BodyLogic

Enjoy your journey!

Ian + Melanie

BodyLogic

**How to customize your healthy lifestyle
by focusing on *gains,* not losses**

BodyLogic LLC

Manufactured in the United States of America

Library of Congress Catalog Card Number: 97-95336

ISBN: 0-9662050-0-6

Cartoons: Ralph Smith

Cover design: Pearl and Associates

Book design and production by Tabby House

BodyLogic LLC

15 NE 181 St. Ave.
Portland, OR 97230-6659
E-mail: BodyLo1997@aol.com
www.BodyLogic-Is-For-Me.com

Dedication

We lovingly dedicate this book to our family, who loved us so much it hurt. Though you brought us pain, we thank you for unknowingly giving us the courage to live, the strength to change, and the power to overcome life's challenges and injustices.

Thank you! We love you!

The Child Is The Family...

They are the mirror images of you,
Their bodies and souls once nourished by food.
In the pain you brought they found their way,
These children of the past are now women today.

The pain it gave them strength to grow,
Through the direction you gave, they found their road.
These children of the past are women of wealth,
Their lives now nourished by love of self.

Melonie Heaton

Important Notice—Please Read:

This book makes no attempt to prescribe any diet or exercise plan. BodyLogic is not a diet. It is a way of life that you discover, customize and implement by yourself, for yourself.

The reader is advised to consult a physician or other health-care professional prior to beginning any new food, activity or health program to make sure the program is appropriate for your individual needs. If you have a history of, or suspect any mental health disorders, you should consult with a licensed mental health professional before beginning any program that addresses emotional problems. The authors and the publisher disclaim liability for any adverse effects from the use of application of the information contained in this book. While this book describes a food, activity and health improvement program, it is based upon personal experiences and is not intended to be a prescription. No guarantes of benefit are made from the application of the information contained in this book. The information contained in this book is not provided as medical advice. Through the distribution of this publication, the authors submit they are not engaged in rendering health care, medical or dietary advice. If health-care, medical or dietary services are required, you should seek the advice of your physical or mental health-care providers.

The authors and the publisher disclaim all liability for any loss, damage, injury or expense caused arising from the reliance upon or application of any information provided in this book and do not warrant the truth, accuracy or completeness of the information provided. The authors assume no responsibility for the accuracy contained herein. Although the authors have researched all sources to ensure the accuracy and completeness of the information contained in this book, they assume no responsibility for errors, inaccuracies, omissions or any other inconsistency herein. Any slights against people or organizations are unintentional.

The Road To BodyLogic

Introduction

*Give your body what it needs, when it needs it, and
your body will take care of the rest. That's BodyLogic!
Trash that diet before it trashes you!*

Have you ever noticed that the word "diet" is actually the word "die"
with the letter "t" added to it? Diets kill. Diets destroy your mind and
body. Think about that one!

Here's more food for thought. Look at the word "fatal." You got it:
fat will kill you!

After twenty-five years plus of medical research, the "experts" have
failed to come up with a solution for "fatness." We discovered why
the answer has been so elusive. The experts have not been looking
at the obvious! The solution is not in a magic food, supplement or a
miracle drug. The answer is not in the genes. The answer is not
necessarily in the food that you do or do not eat! There is no "one-
size-fits-all" when it comes to finding the solution for fatness. The
answers are within you! Being fat is the result of a lack of balance
between the mind and the body! Your perception of being fat is a
reflection of what is on the inside. Make the choice to listen to your
mind and body, and give them what they need. It's that simple. That's
BodyLogic!

Not convinced yet? Would you believe it if a physician who lived
from 460–370 B.C. was one of the first to touch on this basic concept?
Ever heard of Hippocrates? He was a Greek physician, recognized as
the father of medicine. He believed that disease results from an imbalance in the body, and this imbalance should be treated with diet
and hygiene. In our minds, Hippocrates was half right. He didn't take
into account the powerful influence of the mind! Physicians of our
time take the Hippocratic Oath. Hippocrates did not develop the
oath, but modern medicine is based on the principles of Hippocrates.

It's no wonder the experts have not been able to find the solution for fatness! They are still thinking like Hippocrates did long ago! They have not considered the uniqueness of each body, mind and soul.

Forget everything you have ever read, every diet you have ever tried and all of the current hype about food, exercise and weight loss. We will explain to you, our opinion of the true relationship between food and body weight.

BodyLogic will provide you with the tools to customize your own personal lifestyle change. Your body is unlike any other. Why be forced into a "canned" program that may not work for you? Diet foods and structured diets make you sick and fat! Look inside to find the choices that are right for you!

Being "overfat" and "overweight" are not the same thing. You can be "overfat" and healthy! You can be "overweight" and healthy. By changing your lifestyle and self esteem, you will begin to accomplish more than you ever set out to do.

This book is written for the 180-pound-plus woman who chooses to return her body to a state of balance. The concepts are adaptable to almost anyone of any age, weight or sex who wants to improve how they feel. This book is not just about losing fat! It is about adding quality years to your life, and quality life to your years!

Most of the books on the market today are geared toward the ten- to fifteen-pound loser without taking into consideration the other factors that make you a person! Most of us have feelings of anger, hate, hurt, resentment, betrayal, etc. to be resolved. We are pro-grammed to diminish stress through the use of food, whether it be overeating, compulsive dieting or binging and purging. With time and development of new habits, you will learn to gain control of those things in your life that are within your power to control. You will come to the understanding that food is your fuel, not a substitute for comfort, security or love!

The French dramatist Molière (1622–73) delivered the message in *The Miser:* "One should eat to live, not live to eat."

There is no right and wrong, good or bad, when it comes to you and your food. There is only choice. Food, self-exploration, moving your body and making the commitment to change are choices. Your weight is a destination, not a destiny.

Being fat is the result of the choices you make. Once you begin to accept and live this concept, fat loss may occur almost effortlessly.

Begin your new life today by looking into the mirror and realizing that the reflection staring back at you is your past. Climb on the scale, record the number, write it down, then write this down: "The number means nothing. The scale is my enemy. The scale is like a cult, it controls me. The scale allows me to approve or disapprove of myself each time I hesitantly climb onto it."

From here on, you will be measuring gains, not losses, and weight will no longer be the focus of your attention or obsession.

Starting a new life and really living it is the most wonderful and enjoyable gift you can ever give yourself. It is a lifelong journey. Have fun along the way. Before you begin, empty your suitcase of that old diet mentality and dump it in the trash along with your scale. Never again be attached to the umbilical cord of a scale!

From here on, your wellness will be measured by the way you feel physically and emotionally. It will be measured by the way your clothes fit, and by the way your body fits into a chair, airline seat, bathtub or shower stall. Ultimately, your wellness will be measured by the inspiration you give to others.

Your authors are women. Therefore, you will find many stories and examples that relate to women. However, we recognize that men have many of the same issues and in many ways are similarly discriminated against because of their weight and perceived health. We provide valuable information for male readers as well. The words "diet" and "exercise" are used as descriptive terms only. From here on out, your thoughts should be focused on getting well!

The concept of BodyLogic was developed by Melonie Heaton, out of sheer determination to improve her own health after a lifetime of poor habits. She lost eighty-five pounds by making some simple changes in the way she lives. Melonie is living proof that BodyLogic works for her! Your co-author, Jan Heaton, is just beginning her own journey toward a healthier life. You will follow Jan as her lifestyle change develops. She will give you candid comments and progress reports.

It is our firm belief that making the changes necessary to achieve wellness is much easier if you know what to expect. We have "been there, done that." Our goal is not to put you on a "diet." Our goal is to teach you the concepts behind BodyLogic, and support you as you experience your own journey.

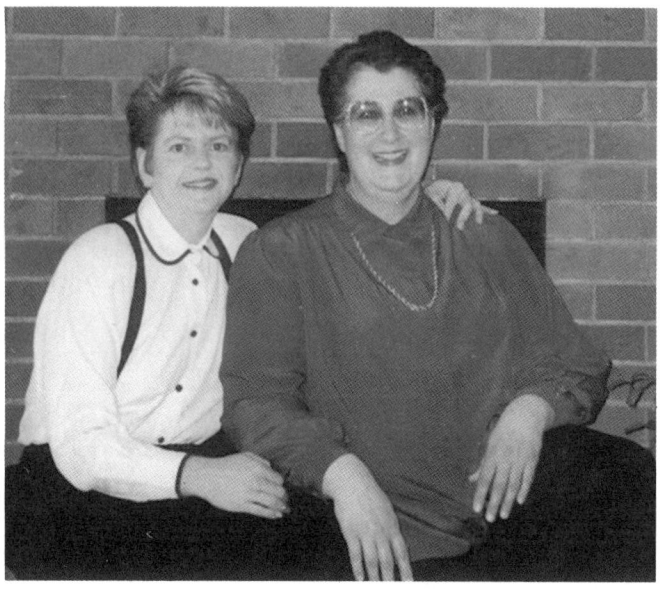

Your BodyLogic guides, Melonie (left), and Jan Heaton

The future is up to you and is a result of the choices you make. ***Don't Die-It, Live-It!***

> ***Your positive self statement for today: "I believe in me."***
>
> "It is possible to believe that all the past is but the beginning of a beginning, and that all that is and has been is but the twilight of the dawn. It is possible to believe that all the human mind has ever accomplished is but the dream before the awakening."
>
> —*H. G. Wells (1866–1946), British author, "The Discovery of the Future," Lecture, 24 Jan. 1902, at the Royal Institute, London (published in* Nature, *no. 65, 1902).*

Reflections

I look in the mirror and who do I see?
A huge, fat woman staring back at me.
I ask of myself, "But how can this be?"
My measurements reflect much less than I see.
My eyes are my mirror ... They tell the story...
My fat was my armor, to protect me from pain,
My courage overshadowed by fears of gain.
Fears of success, beauty and love,
Were comforted by fat, like a fleece-lined glove.
A fat baby, a fat child, a fat teen, a fat woman.
"Why should such pain be imposed on this human?"
"Is my reflection what it appears?"
The image I see is the experience of my years.
Always a misfit, always the last,
The woman of my present is the child of my past.
Food strengthened my armor, it provided safety and nurture.
Food is my life, my past and my future.
My eyes are my mirror, they tell the story...
One day came alone and depressed,
I realized my life was a heck of a mess!
A decision must be made, to live or to die.
I wept and I ate, then looked in my eyes.
The answer it appeared, it was there all along.
This woman had the courage to be strong!
To have control in my life was the key,
I am not FAT, it is FAT that is ME!

A new sense of strength, a brand new me,
The tide of my past went out like the sea.
Old issues examined then buried for good,
My armor no longer came from my food.
Balance became the focus of attention.
To be skinny and fit no longer my obsession
I cared for myself with love and affection
My mind and body built their connection.
The child of my present, is the woman of my future...
I look in the mirror and who do I see?
An ever growing woman smiling back at me.
My body HAD changed! My vision had cleared.
The woman in the mirror IS what she appears!
Their eyes are a mirror, they tell the story...
I look in their eyes and what do I see?
Reflections of desire flow in, like the tide of the sea.
"How does she do it? Willpower it must be!"
"Not power of will, the power of me!"
"The answer is simple," I further explain.
"I choose to fuel my fire, not extinguish my flame."
In touch with my body, I know what it knows.
I listen and respond. I no longer fear food.
Their eyes are my mirror, they tell the story...
Our choice is forever to continue this journey.
Whether to fuel the fire or extinguish the flame?
The choices we make reflect our gains.
The child of my present is the woman of my future.
This new life will thrive, with constant care and nurture.

Melonie Heaton

Part One

Fine-Tune That Engine

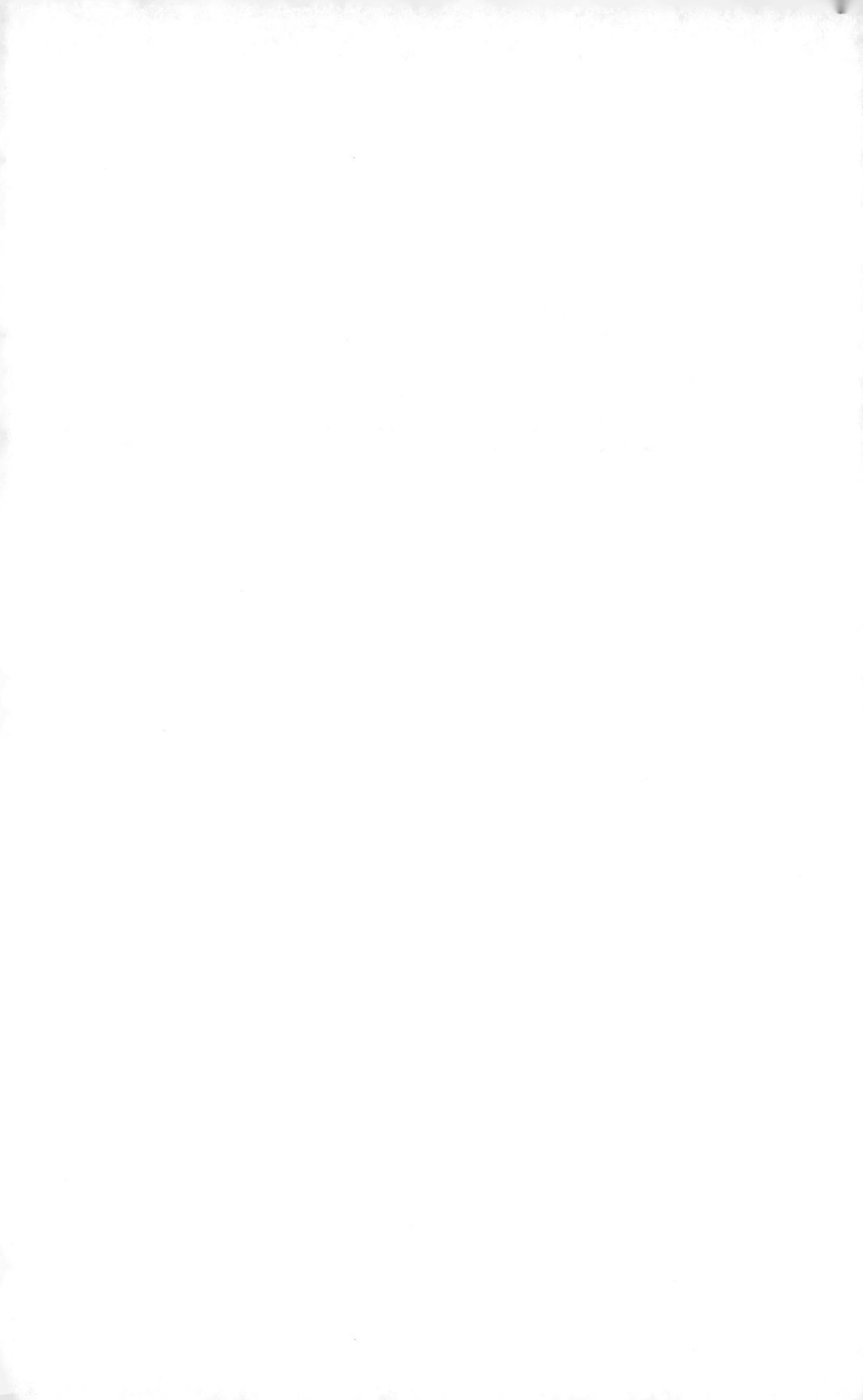

BodyLogic 101

Learn It, Live It, Share It, Inspire It

"Obesity is not a disease, an inherited trait or a destiny. It is a destination." —Melonie Heaton, RN

One Sunday morning, I was leisurely sipping coffee, procrastinating about getting up and about. Nothing was on TV. The morning news was quite depressing. I unconsciously began channel surfing. Within fifteen minutes, I stumbled upon at least four segments on different channels discussing various types of diets, why some work and why some don't. My feathers really became ruffled.

One segment was an infommercial, with two physicians talking about how their weight-loss program was the best to come about in years, that it is the only one that "works." After listening a bit, I discovered it was nothing more than a high-protein, moderate-fat, low-carbohydrate diet. It is the very type of diet that has made many of us lose weight and then gain it back with some to spare, while feeling sick in the process.

Physicians, of all people, promoting this kind of destruction to the human body! Really, to come on the air and only tell part of the facts. These physicians said that carbohydrates all turn into sugar once digested, and then the sugar is converted and stored as fat. The premise being if you don't eat carbohydrates (we will refer to them as "carbs" or "carbos"), you won't gain weight. They neglected to mention that glucose (the kind of sugar you get when carbos are digested) is the body's chief fuel source, and the major fuel source used by the brain and nervous tissue. Sounds to me, according to this theory, if you stop eating so many carbs, you will be thin, but likely you will be brain dead as well. Some trade-off, huh? (I do have to be fair. Carbohydrates not used for immediate energy are converted and stored as fat.)

Another script, this one part of the local news health segment, revealed that the latest research shows low-fat diets don't work, that we should be consuming mono and polyunsaturated fats and avoiding hydrogenated and most animal fats. The view is that "good" fats lower LDL (bad cholesterol) and raise HDL (good cholesterol). OK, I can buy that, at least the part about good and bad fats. However, fat is still fat! Too much of it makes you fat.

You know what? Here are some real fat facts in which you can sink your teeth. Low-fat diets don't work. High-protein, low-carbohydrate diets don't work. High-carbohydrate, low-protein diets don't work. High-fat diets definitely do not work, and low-calorie diets do not work. *No diets work, ladies and gentlemen!* Diets deprive the body of what it needs to function. The definition of a diet is restriction of food, or restriction of fuel. How far will your car run on an empty gas tank? How long will your gas barbecue work if the propane tank is nearly empty? How long will your portable stereo play on dead batteries? The same concepts hold true for the human body.

You know what else really makes me angry? It's how all of these scientists, researchers and nutritionists seem to think they can tell the rest of us what the magic fix is for obesity! There is no magic fix. There is no magic pill. Lord knows the researchers have tried, and just when they thought they had the magic pill, they find out it kills some of us. How do they know what works for *you* and *me* if we were not part of their so called research studies?

I *know* what works for me. BodyLogic will teach you to learn what works for you. This book is not about diets. I said it before and I will say it again. I will keep saying it: *Diets destroy your mind and body!* Sure, you may lose "weight" for awhile, but likely you will gain it back and then some. The weight you lose may not be fat. Yet the weight that comes back most likely will be fat! We explain why.

Having a healthy body is not necessarily about losing weight. It is about making a few simple changes in how you live, to reprogram your body to lose fat. How much fat you lose is up to you, and your body's own desire. Part of this you can influence, part of it you can't. You can be overfat and healthy. This book is not about starvation, or killing yourself at the gym. It is not entirely focused on psychology.

This book is about a logical, common-sense approach to achieving wellness.

This book is written by real women, for real women (and men, too). We talk to you as if we were face to face. Real women do not diet. Real women teach their minds to manage their bodies. That is the basic concept behind BodyLogic. It's that simple.

Too good to be true, you may ask? You know what they say, if something sounds too good to be true, it probably is. BodyLogic is simple, but it's not easy. It takes a lot of hard work to overcome years of abusing your body through diets and improper exercise programs. Yes, food and exercise are critical to health, but you will find very little structure to BodyLogic. It is not expected that everything we write in this book should be taken literally. We give you the tools to change your lifestyle. That means making small changes in the way you eat and move your body. More importantly, BodyLogic teaches you how to unleash the power of your mind. That is where true success begins.

You have had it inside of you all along. You have the answers, though you may not be aware of them just yet. BodyLogic will help you uncover the answers hidden deep inside of your brain, the answers that will move you toward a state of optimum health and wellness, no matter what your body size is. While there is nothing funny about being overfat, we do use a lot of humor as we talk to you. Laughter is the best medicine of all.

The first chapter or two may sound quite serious in many respects. They are. These are the very personal stories of your authors. You likely will be able to relate to our stories and our struggles, because "we have been there, done that." We do know what and how you feel, because we *have* been there, and in many ways are still there.

Our biggest frustration with the myriad so-called "diet" and "weight-loss" books out there is that we are unable to relate to them from the first page on. They are often written by people who have never had a "real" weight problem in their lives. Anyone can tweak their food intake to lose ten or fifteen pounds, but pounds of what? Fat? Muscle? Water? They force you to eat things that are just plain "weird," things you don't routinely have around the house and often things you really don't like. How can you make positive changes that last a lifetime if you hate every change you make? Who should your role models be? In our opinion, not some celebrity whose scale never read above 160. To think you can combine certain foods, totally avoid others, or live entirely on vegetables, beans and brown rice and lose all the fat you want, is impossible and unrealistic.

BodyLogic is possible. It is realistic. BodyLogic teaches you to make realistic changes and achieve realistic goals. You will succeed in your own way, and at your own pace.

We would bet money that you are much like us. You gave up dieting long ago, for fear of yet another failure and of regaining your weight. You decided to stop dieting for the deprivation, both physically and mentally, you would feel during the process. You may have come to the conclusion that it is better to be fat and healthy than skinny and sick! Just one major problem for many of us is this: We are both fat and sick! We can't seem to find the answer. We live our lives doing for others, to guarantee a circle of friends. It does not matter how much we are used during the process. It does not matter how much we neglect our own needs either. Our lives are spent seeking acceptance in any way we can find it. If you have been overfat all of your life, it's likely we may have hit a home run here!

Have you begun to realize there is something terribly wrong with this picture? Are you allowing people, food and things to control both your mind and your body? Their interactions with you control you. Food controls you by providing things that are otherwise missing in your life, like love, security and satisfaction. It is the lack of control over your own life that makes you a fat person on the outside. It is your role models and life experiences growing up that will keep you a fat person on the inside no matter how much you reduce the size of your body. We will explain later why this is such a positive thing.

Here is an eye opener for you. Read back a couple of paragraphs, where we suggested that you may have given up dieting for fear of the mental and physical deprivation that would likely result. Bingo! You have the answer staring you right in the face. You likely have figured out from firsthand experience that diets do not work, but you may not know the reason why. Many of us live every minute of every day in fear of food. What we fear intensely we think about constantly. To overcome this fear, you must give yourself permission to eat! You must believe that food nourishes your body and your brain. Your relationship with food is what makes you fat.

This book is not about dieting. In fact, after you have read the first few chapters, we will once again ask you to toss your scale in the trash and never purchase another.

This book is about regaining control of your life. This book is about health. It is about physical and emotional wellness. It is not just about losing weight. If your only goal is to lose "weight," you are not yet ready for BodyLogic. If you say you cannot find even thirty minutes in each day to really care for yourself, then you are not yet ready to make the kind of commitment that will last a lifetime. If various types of poor quality food are more important to you than your health, then you are not ready to make the commitment to change. We firmly believe that it is better to be overfat and healthy, rather than to diet and be sick. However, one lovely benefit of BodyLogic, if incorporated into your life rather than just practiced, is fat loss. (There is a difference between "fat" loss and "weight" loss!) It would be very difficult to live your life through BodyLogic and not lose at least some fat. We consider the fat loss that results from BodyLogic to be icing on the cake, or "dessert," so to speak! We say this because it happens as a result of the changes you make in your life, not some ridiculous diet on which you put yourself.

Diets don't work. Diets kill. Diets starve your body of the nutrition it needs to live in a healthy way. Diets control your mind. Diets ruin your body and your spirit. Diets are just plain stupid!

BodyLogic requires no strict food or exercise plans. It requires no expensive nutritional supplements. You eat *real* food. (Note: The focus here is on the word "real.") You eat as much as you need, and the kinds of "real" food that you like. If you are like us, you are probably thinking to yourself, *How many other diet books have I read that statement in, and found it to be just the opposite?* The difference is this. BodyLogic is not a diet. It is a way of life. BodyLogic is individualized. It is a process you do yourself, for yourself, to find a lifestyle that is healthy for *you*. BodyLogic is many small changes over time. You will never be asked to force yourself into someone else's plan ever again. One size does not fit all. It's true for clothes, and it's true for diets. That's one reason diets don't work, never have and never will.

Think of it this way. Look at animals in the wild. They have no social pressures to be thin, or beautiful. They do not wear clothes. Strength is important for survival. Wild animals eat when hungry, drink when thirsty, and they eat and drink what they need, as long as they can find it. Wild animals rest very little. They almost appear to be in a constant state of motion, whether it be meandering about looking for food, or running or fighting for survival. They instinctively know what food they should eat, and which foods kill. They function on instinct. How many overfat coyotes, wolves or deer have you seen? Sure, bears put on fat as they go into hibernation for the winter, but they awake much thinner in the spring. This is a survival mechanism to prevent the bears from starving to death in the winter. Our early ancestors lived much the same way, but unfortunately, our bodies did not change their instincts as society came to be what it is today. Our problem as a human race is this: We have stopped listening to our instincts, in lieu of enjoying all of today's conveniences. The answer to the problem is simple: We relearn old instincts, and adapt them to the conveniences and technology of today.

BodyLogic reteaches the brain to control the body the way nature had originally intended. At first, BodyLogic will not be easy. But it is simple. Think of a child learning to walk. Learning this new skill is full of challenges, but once mastered and incorporated into the child's set of skills, it becomes effortless. The child walks without even thinking about it. It is the same way with any new skill one learns. At first it takes focus and practice. Once mastered, it is second nature.

Let's look at some definitions for a moment:

1. Body: the physical structure of a person or animal.

2. Logic: the mind functioning in a reasonable, sound, intelligent manner.

Most of us at one time or another have heard of the amazing power of the mind to control what happens to the body. Humans can will themselves to live, or they can will themselves to die. The more powerful the desire, the more the mind is able to control the body. By purchasing this book, you have indicated the desire to change something about the way in which you live your life. Body-Logic is the ultimate gift you could ever give to yourself.

Here's a progress report on Jan. It took her only two weeks to reduce her total daily fat intake from about 60 percent to 30 percent, (a much healthier level) all by replacing Half & Half with whole milk and replacing margarine with a quality substitute. She still eats three beef hot dogs for lunch! "I love the butter goop! I can't believe it's this easy!" said Jan.

As you read this book, you will learn the process of BodyLogic. We will give you the tools you need to achieve whatever goals you may have. The choice to use the tools we provide is yours! The choice to make a commitment to improve your life and your health is yours. BodyLogic is nothing but your own choices! You choose the foods you will eat and in what quantities. You choose how and when to move your body. Can you see any deprivation in all of those choices? From here on out, please focus on what you wish to gain, not what you wish to lose. The mind is a powerful thing. It can either heal or destroy. Learn to listen to it. Learn to control it! Establish the connection between your body and your mind. That's BodyLogic!

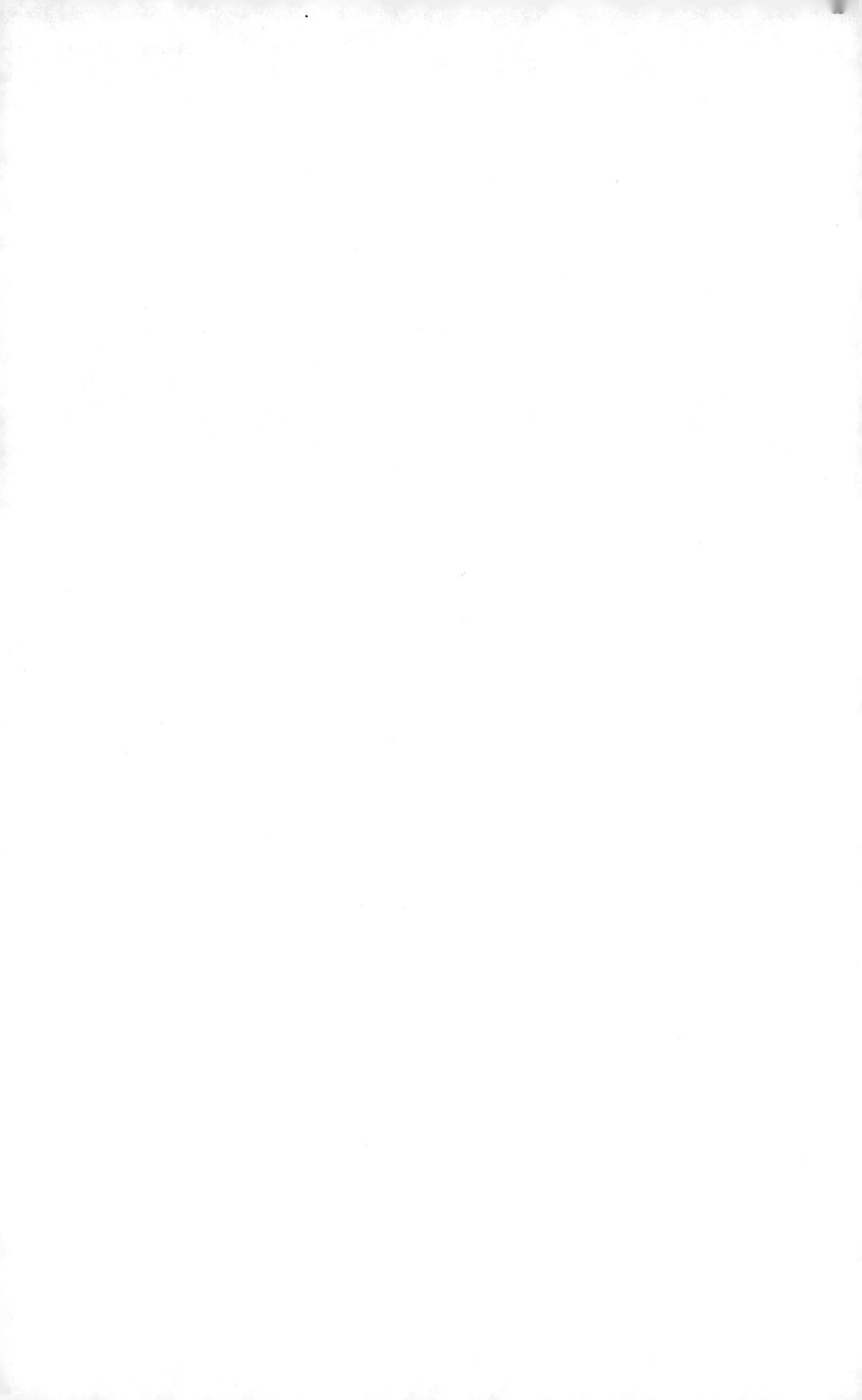

The Model "M"

Melonie's Story

I have always been a very private person. For the first time in my life I have found the strength and courage to share my innermost thoughts and feelings with complete strangers. This is not out of some need for self-fulfillment, but to show you through my experiences that I have "been there, done that." I understand what you are going through. Though I cannot be there personally to support you through the wonderfully difficult but enriching days ahead, I do hope that you will refer to this book often for encouragement. When you have met your personal goal, you will become an inspiration to others. Give something back by giving a copy of this book to a friend or someone you care about. (Keep your copy to read again and again for inspiration and support.) Better yet, help that person embark on their own journey toward wellness.

My story is not shared as a way to gain your pity. It is not intended to depress you. It is provided as an example of how we become the people we are, for better or for worse. In order to know where you are going, you must first realize and accept where you have been. I firmly believe that obesity is a destination. It is not a disease, an inherited trait or a destiny. An overfat person is a product of the environment in which he or she is raised. This environment often teaches us that food is the center of social activities, that physical activity is a negative. In other words, for many of us our role models have taught that food is comfort, pleasure and safety. Our role models often teach us that physical activity is the cause of discomfort, injury and displeasure. These lessons are often taught unknowingly.

To this day I continue to reflect on my childhood and discover more reasons why I became the person I am. Memories are recalled through discussions with friends and family. While writing this book, my co-author (who is also my cousin) and I have had the opportunity to get to really know each other. She has played an important role in helping me to further understand who I really am. I am the product of loving family and friends. However, through their style of loving, they instilled in me a negative self-image about my spirit and my body which haunts me still today. In order to be successful at changing any one part of your lifestyle, you must come to an understanding of how you adopted your original lifestyle in the first place.

The Evolution of the Model "M"

I was brought up in a middle-class family, with a mother and father, and a brother. I cannot remember a time that I ever wanted for anything as far as material things go. There was always plenty of food, toys to play with, a bike, braces, music lessons and money to do things with my friends every weekend. Family gatherings, holidays and even quiet weekends at home were always centered around food. I was always fat.

(Yes, I am using the "F" word. As we are all in this together, let's not play games and hide behind "nice," "politically correct" words. The first step in changing your lifestyle is to really see who you are today, and who you want to be tomorrow.)

My earliest memory is that of a fat four-year-old child. I remember my mother lovingly trying to put me on diet after diet. I vividly remember seeking out friends who had an unlocked kitchen, so to speak. I would seek out snacks at other people's homes. I remember my mother talking to me about such food-seeking behavior, and I remember feeling ashamed. My mother was one of those people who could not keep enough weight on, always eating whatever she wanted. She loved her desserts and whole cream on her cereal, and butter or margarine on everything. She never exercised. My mother was not one to show much affection through hugging or spending quality time with me. When I was a child, my mother and I were never very close.

As I grew into adulthood, I realized that she obtained some inner satisfaction from having such powerful control over me. She did love me, and she showed it through maintaining an exquisitely clean home, hot meals on the table and through trying to control my food intake. She would ration my portions and forbid me to drink soda pop or eat candy. Halloween was the exception. My bag of goodies was placed on the top shelf of the pantry. I was allowed one piece per day, while the rest of the family would dive into my bag freely, when they thought I was not looking.

My father was the exact opposite of my mother in many ways. He was the overweight, loving teddy-bear type. He traveled a lot on business and routinely was home only on the weekends. Occa-

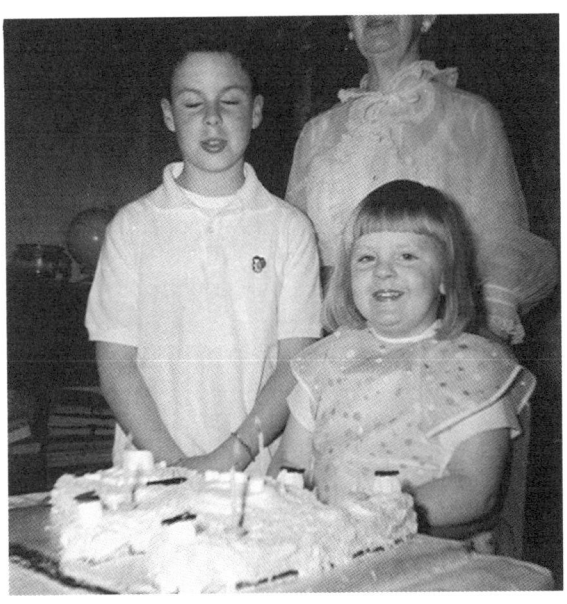

Melonie Heaton at age four. The beginning of her diet roller-coaster ride that lasted thirty years.

sionally he would leave the country for months at a time. I remember many father-daughter weekends, where I would go to his office with him and then out to lunch. We would shop for Christmas or birthdays together. Often we would curl up on the sofa to watch football on TV, and of course, munch on cheese and crackers, salami, popcorn, chips, Christmas candy, nuts, or any number of other such snacks. At that age, I didn't care about football, and didn't understand a thing about the game. For me, football meant love, safety and nurturing. Perhaps you can see how my father taught me to seek comfort in food.

I will not mention my brother very often as we were never close. In fact, I could not stand him. He physically and emotionally abused me from the time I was about five years old. At least that is my earliest recollection. Much of the abuse I suppressed until after the death of my parents. At first thought I was not going to mention him at all, but in order to understand why I grew up fat, I had to face everything that happened while I was growing up. My brother was six years older than I. He was thin, very active, and always getting into trouble. He picked on me constantly, and as I understand now, manipulated me mentally and physically so that I would lie for him when he did something wrong. He constantly got into trouble, whether it was by skipping school, shoplifting, stealing the family car, or committing some of his many other crimes which only worsened in severity as he got older. He would of course be the one to get all of my parents' attention, leaving me to hide in my bedroom, listening to the screaming, crying, and eating myself silly from the stash of goodies I hid under my bed. I would sneak out on the weekends and go to the convenience store down the street. This is where I would spend my allowance on candy. That became the stash under my bed, and the start of my closet-eating behavior.

My father's career demanded that the family relocate frequently. By the time I started college, I had moved thirteen times. The longest we stayed in any one city was five years, and the shortest nine months. Often, we would move during the summer. When I was very young, I made friends easily. All the neighborhood kids would gather around the moving van when we moved in. Instant friends! I was a very active young child, swimming every day during the summer. I loved long bike rides, roller skating and ice skating. Occasionally, the family would go bowling on Sunday mornings. We would always come home and eat steak and eggs for brunch afterwards. Sunday dinners were a tradition. My father loved to cook and the fare was usually homemade fried chicken and french fries.

At about the age of six, I vividly recall getting sick to my stomach with vomiting and severe stomach cramps every Monday afternoon. Sometimes this would hit after my noon meal and I would have to come home early. I would also get terrible headaches. The only thing that would help would be to go to bed and sleep. After several months of this, my parents became concerned and took me to the family doctor, who found nothing wrong other than my weight. He suggested that I was overtired from playing too hard on the weekend. From that day forward, I was banned from playing with my friends or engaging in any strenuous physical activity on Sundays. Through discussions with my cousin, Jan, I came to the realization that this was the first time the concept of physical activity being a negative thing was instilled in me.

My cousin also suggested that perhaps school was a negative for me, and illness was my way of escaping an uncomfortable experience and getting more attention from my family. The more I reflect on this concept, the more certain I am that this is the case.

School was never a positive place for me. Though I always earned excellent grades, I was constantly picked on by other kids, often getting hit and teased about my weight. In those days, girls had to wear dresses to school, and of course the boys loved to lift up those dresses to take a peek at what was underneath. In addition, I was quite shy. I dreaded days when I had to read out loud in class or do any sort of public speaking. If I knew of these situations in advance, I would become so anxious that I would make myself sick. Of course, as soon as I got home, the illness would disappear!

As I got older, it became harder and harder to make friends, and I would literally eat my summers away until fall when I would start school and slowly make new friends, only to find myself moving in a year or two and having to do it all over again. I think a point in my life came when it was less painful to be alone, than it was to make friends and have to leave them. I remember avoiding gym class, as I would always be teased about my weight and lack of physical ability. The school showers after gym were the worst. I was so embarrassed. I felt all the more alone, a fat girl on a skinny-girls-only-island. I never enjoyed physical activity after that.

From my earliest days, I remember using food to fill a void, whether it be the frequent absences of my father, the food restrictions of my mother, the loneliness or the pain my brother brought to our family. It seems clear now—I used food to replace the physical and emotional gestures of love and the need to belong that my life was lacking.

Life never seemed to get any easier. After I became a teenager, my father's health began to fail. He had several serious health problems, mostly related to his lifetime of smoking, moderate drinking, eating high-fat foods and leading a sedentary lifestyle. His work-life was a pressure cooker, and he looked far beyond his fifty-six years when he died.

My brother had begun his own destructive lifestyle years before. He dropped out of school, and associated with the wrong crowd. He was in trouble with the law, used drugs and alcohol, and had just finished one of many jail sentences when my father died. My brother had recently married a woman who used drugs, and had a three-year-old daughter by another marriage.

My father died in May of my sixteenth year, and only a month later I went to Sun Valley, Idaho, to work as a housekeeper for the summer, my first time away from home. This summer had been planned for many months, and while I did not want to leave my mother alone, she insisted. Her health began to take a slow, downward turn at that point; she battled pneumonia right after the death of my father. By the end of summer, she had recovered from that, and continued her part-time job at a dry-cleaning establishment she had started the winter before.

Life went fairly smoothly for the next year and a half. My brother never lived at home again, but continued to get into trouble, and had tried to commit suicide on several occasions. Each time he would upset my mother, she would stop eating and I would double mine. High school graduation day came. I don't think my mother was ever more proud. After the death of my father, my mother and I became very, very close.

The summer following my graduation, my mother and I moved about sixty miles away so I could attend college. We decided to share an apartment, rather than me going to live in a dorm, to keep expenses down. My mother started work at the university library, made many good friends and finally began to feel somewhat whole again. Four years later, I graduated from nursing school and moved some seventy-five miles away to go to work at a small-town hospital as there were no jobs available in our community. After six months, I moved back home with my mother—my work hours were not guaranteed and I could not make ends meet. I had spent those long days of summer not working much, but eating constantly.

I worked at a local hospital for the next three and a half years, mostly nights. My mother worked days so we rarely saw each other. I lost about forty pounds working a very active night nursing job.

During this time, I also became obsessed with my weight, trying every diet known. As my mother and I rarely ate together, it was much easier for me to control what I ate. The forty pounds came off with a low-carbohydrate, high-protein diet, but not without a price. I began to feel terrible. I had no energy, had frequent headaches and became quite irritable. Sleeping was impossible. I went off that diet and regained the forty pounds, plus twenty more for good measure. I then continued to try every diet in every woman's magazine. I tried more diet books than I can remember. I didn't stay with any of them. I would lose a few pounds, then I would have all those same symptoms and feel totally deprived and depressed. As soon as I would go off whatever diet I had been on, I would regain what I had lost, always with ten or twenty additional pounds.

At age twenty-six, I took a management job out of state. It was at that time I realized how much our mother-daughter roles had changed. I was no longer the child, but the substitute for my father. I took on many of the household duties that my father always had done. My mother never wanted to increase her independence. Even the simple things such as fixing a leaking faucet or gassing up the car at the self-serve island became my responsibility. I took care of all of the outside chores, mowing the lawn in summer and shoveling snow in winter. I even took over most of the cooking at some point. I became my mother's husband in many ways, and soon came to the belief that she needed me to take care of her. My mother quit her library job and moved out of state with me, much due to my own insistence. I could not stand having her all alone six hundred miles away. That was probably the biggest mistake of my life. My mother chose to retire a few years early. She was never one to socialize with other women, or participate in community service projects. She had no hobbies, no interests outside of work and cleaning house. She became a hermit, and relied on me more than ever for her social life and to fulfill her emotional needs. As I know now, part of her emotional needs were filled through her control over me.

Six months after the move, she had a heart attack and nearly died. I woke up in the middle of the night and heard strange noises coming from her room. I found her unresponsive, thrashing about in bed. She had torn her nightgown to shreds from all of the thrashing. I called 911 and she was rushed to the hospital, suffering seizures from the lack of oxygen to her brain. She spent three days in intensive care, not knowing who I was. In a way, this ordeal was a blessing, forcing her into a diet and exercise program. She began walking, stopped smoking and began to eat a low-salt, low-fat diet, all of which she hated.

Unfortunately, her near-death experience did not encourage me to change my lifestyle. Again, she was my role model, showing me that when someone is forced into a "diet" or "exercise" program, they feel deprived and out of control. My mother hated having to give up the foods she loved. It's no wonder she didn't stick with it long.

I ate what she ate when at home, but splurged on all of those now "forbidden" foods while I was at work. And I worked long days, often twelve to sixteen hours. I worried constantly about my mother, and was obsessed with worry about her dying. The more I worried, the more I ate. I soon reached my maximum weight, topping 225 pounds for my 5' 4" frame.

A year and a half later, I took another job 1,300 miles away in Seattle. As my mother and I were both born in Washington, and all of our family was there, we were elated to be moving home. My new job resulted in a pay cut, which combined with the higher cost of living forced my mother and me once again into sharing an apartment. We shared all of the expenses, but yet again I took care of my mother. She made no effort to make friends, or get involved in any activities. She then was diagnosed with possible cancer, and had a hysterectomy. She recovered well from the surgery, but never fully resumed her walking program, and she started smoking again. This all led to her falling back into her old eating habits, though cream on her cereal was now a weekly treat, rather than a daily habit.

Meanwhile, my brother had divorced, had a child with a woman he did not marry, left that woman, served several more jail terms, then died from a drug and alcohol overdose. My brother's death broke my mother's heart. Though she did not approve of the life he had led, he was still her son and she loved him.

A year later, I changed jobs again, and we moved some thirty miles away so I would not have to commute. We moved to the same town where I had attended junior high. My mother had a few friends there and saw them often, which made her much happier. She began walking more consistently, and starting paying more attention to eating healthier foods. Again I did not follow her lead. I had given up on ever losing weight after all of those years of yo-yo dieting. My high-stress job and long work hours left no time and no desire to exercise or eat right. Another two years flew by. My mother's health had waxed and waned. She began to lose a lot of weight, and felt ill most of the time. I could see she was getting depressed. The more her health failed, the more stressed I became, and the more I ate.

My mother died that same year. Years of arthritis, smoking, stress, poor diet and lack of exercise had taken its toll. I became even more depressed and withdrawn, having lost my best friend. For a month or so after that, I fought the urge to end my own life. I had nothing left to live for, or so I thought. After several months, through the support of my family and friends, my depression began to lift, though I missed my mother terribly. I spent quiet time eating to make myself feel better.

I threw myself back into my work, and filled the void of having lost my mother by working even harder, and eating more and more. I changed jobs yet again another year later. I was very happy in my new position and had many friends, but still felt something was missing in my life. I felt awful all of the time. I was fat and exhausted. I would go into the office at 6:30 A.M. not feeling rested after ten hours of sleep. My days were soon filled with the same routine. Up at 5:00 A.M., breakfast, to work by 6:30 A.M., a snack of cookies at 10:00 A.M., lunch at 11:30 A.M., and total exhaustion by 2:00 P.M. More cookies for a pick-me-up. I found I could not concentrate and would start to doze off at my desk. I would then say I was going home to work, yet another excuse to cover up the way I was feeling physically and emotionally. I would be home by 3:00 P.M., and immediately fall asleep on the couch. I would wake up sometime during "Oprah" then consume some potato chips for dinner, and would usually top that off with ice cream or some other form of chocolate dessert. It was always chocolate. I would fall asleep on the couch again, and wake up at 8:00 P.M., when I would go to bed. The same routine repeated itself for a couple of years.

I'm not quite sure of the exact date when I realized what it was in my life that was missing, and what changes I needed to make if I was to live another ten years. I had lost all of my immediate family due to their own poor health habits, and I did not want to be the next in line. I knew I had a choice: to change my lifestyle or end my life. That is when I first began the journey toward a healthier life. The first major step was realizing that I had lost control of my life. In fact, I don't think I was ever in control of my life. I had spent my entire life caring for others, and obtaining satisfaction and contentment from food. People and food had been in control of me.

The second major step was giving myself permission to put my own needs first, and take care of myself. I put everything else in my life at a lower level of importance. No job, no material things, and no relationships with other people would ever make me happy unless I first was happy with myself. My lifestyle had provided a coat of armor, an excuse not to interact with people so I would never again have to experience the terrible hurt of losing someone I love, or being embarrassed by the comments of insensitive others.

My new life began with the understanding that I am my own best friend, I am successful, I am a good person, and there is a reason why I did not take my own life when I had the desire and opportunity to do so. I was somehow given a second chance to regain control of my life.

With all of my medical knowledge and years of experience teaching others how to lead a healthy lifestyle, I had never really internalized what wellness meant. Trained in a traditional medical environment, I had the belief that wellness was simply the absence of physical disease, and nothing more. I had unconsciously adopted the attitude of "don't do as I do, do as I tell you to do." As a nurse, it was always my first priority to educate others how to take care of themselves. I cared more for my patients than I did for myself.

I did not know what I needed or how to get well. Magazine articles, books, and television programs which focused on health and wellness suddenly became of interest to me. For years, I had considered those topics something other people needed to learn. I knew it all. I was a nurse. I found myself suddenly in the role of the patient, the lay person who needed all of the information I could get my hands on.

I did not just wake up one day and decide to lose weight. I had been there, done that, more times than I could count. I wrote the book on failure. No, I was not going to fall into the diet trap again. I decided I could be fat and improve my health at the same time. I bought no diet books, but I did purchase books that discussed lifestyle change. I bought one exercise book, and tried the program. Just like diets, structured exercise programs don't work. I think one reason is the fact that someone who wants desperately to feel better, will allow the book or program to take control. If you follow such a structured program, you are given few choices to make. Without choice, you are not in control.

Everything I read seemed to have one common theme: "Discover what is eating you, not what you are eating." At first I was in total denial that I had a problem. My weight was hereditary. My father and everyone on his side of the family was overweight. (This was pure denial on my part, as I have known since I was small that I had been adopted.) Certainly my thyroid must not be functioning properly and that is why I was fat. I suddenly had the overwhelming desire to change. The most difficult part of any change is realizing you have a problem and committing yourself to resolving that problem. Once that happened, everything else fell into place naturally. I acknowledged I had a problem because I felt rotten. The review of my life, the self-examination and personal growth, slowly evolved as I began to feel better. In fact, it wasn't until I sat down to write this book that I really began to understand and accept why I am who I am. I use the word "began" because I continue to make new discoveries about my past and myself on a daily basis.

I continue to gain much satisfaction from my career, but I am now in business for myself, having total control of my time and my priorities. With all of the energy I have now, I run two businesses, and until recently also worked a part-time job. I am also attending graduate school. Yet I always find time in my day, at least most days, for self-care. All of the changes I have made have now become as much a part of me as my name. I do count fat grams, carbo grams and protein grams, not to mention calories, but I do it to make sure I am giving my body what it needs, not to become obsessed with how "bad" or "good" I am on any given day. I drive waitresses crazy when I do eat out, with all of my special requests and sometimes strange substitutions. If the establishment will not honor my request, I will either leave or select only coffee or some other beverage and eat later.

What have I learned from this exercise of self exploration? I learned that for me, food and activity are some of the few things in my life I do have control over. I learned that for my entire life, *I had allowed food to control me.* Food provided comfort and pleasure. Once I changed my lifestyle, I came to the realization that food, in its basic form, is fuel and I had much growing to do if I was going to change my relationship with food forever. I still battle that control issue to this day, but it is getting easier.

In the chapters that follow, I will share with you the changes I made, the struggles I had, and what I have achieved. This book is not about providing you with a plan to lose weight, but to give you a road map to develop your own plan for wellness that works for you. It does include some experimentation, but there never will be failure. Once you have made the commitment to yourself to change, you cannot fail. Even one small change for the better is a huge success. Success and wellness cannot be measured in pounds lost, or miles walked. It comes with the satisfaction of knowing you are in control of every part of your life. Healing takes time. The longer you have been mistreating your body, the longer you have been ignoring your own emotional and spiritual needs, the longer it will take to feel good again.

The proof is in the pudding (fat-free, of course!)

A picture is worth a thousand words. Here are my before and after measurements. Keep in mind it took me two and a half years to get to maintenance.

Measurements:	Before:	After:
Chest	41½ inches	33 inches
Bust	45½ inches	34 inches
Under bust	38½ inches	31 inches
Waist	42 inches	27½ inches
Upper hip	50 inches	31 inches
Lower hip	47 inches	34 inches
Right thigh	27 inches	18½ inches
Left thigh	27 inches	18 inches
Right calf	17½ inches	14 inches
Left calf	17½ inches	13¾ inches
Right upper arm	15½ inches	10¾ inches
Left upper arm	15½ inches	10¾ inches
Dress size	22 Woman's	8 Petite

Total inches lost: 108½ inches   Total weight lost: 85½ pounds

Though I consider myself now to be maintaining my lifestyle change, the pounds and inches continue to slowly drop, month after month. At this point, I am very happy with what I have achieved. From here on out, any additional loss of pounds or inches is just icing on the cake, so to speak.

You must want to be healthy more than anything you have ever wanted in your life. You must be willing to make small sacrifices for huge returns. If you are not ready to do that, then read no further. There are no magic cures for a lifetime of inactivity and bad eating habits. Prescription drugs and fad diets only contribute to the problem. You did not put on the pounds overnight. Plan to take as long as necessary to achieve your goals. Make sure your goals are realistic. Set a five-year goal rather than a one-year goal, and make changes that will become effortless in time.

Above all else, give yourself permission to take care of yourself first. Say positive things about yourself and continue to do so on a daily basis. You must begin to love yourself before you can make the changes necessary to get well. There is only one solution for achieving a healthier future. That solution is hiding inside of you. By connecting your body and mind, your health will improve and the fat will slowly disappear. It's that simple. That's BodyLogic!

The Model "J"

Jan's Story

OK, ladies and gentlemen! Have you started your personal inventory? It is highly recommended that you do this, as this is the part of the growth that will be the hardest. Anyone can lose weight, but not all of us can keep it off for two reasons. The first is that the real "issues" have not been resolved. The second is the matter of who controls whom. The body has to be retrained in the process, and told it is no longer in complete control of what happens to it.

The evolution of the Model "J"

I was lucky enough to grow up in one town, with the same house, the same church and with the same circle of friends. We were a family that did things together. We went to church and church camp, the mountains, Sunday rides, family vacations, the beach and our summer lot. We always had that special treat of ice cream on each outing. This is how I learned the association of fun and food going together.

So you ask, what was wrong? We were that familiar dysfunctional family.

I am the youngest of three children. My brothers are four and seven years older than I. My oldest brother remained thin until he married. My younger brother was a pug pot from the time I can ever remember. And I was the same way from the second grade until now. I am fat and have been except for those first seven years of my life.

I, too, as a small child had special times with my father, who is my hero. On Sunday mornings before church, I would sit on his lap facing him and run my hands up his unshaven face and giggle for as long as the game continued. Sunday afternoons were usually spent taking a nap with Dad on the couch in the living room. That was until I became so big that we both did not fit on the couch.

I can remember my second grade teacher asking me, when she was measuring us for height and weight—a common practice the fifties—if I had rocks in my pockets. You see, I had on a dress that had three pockets on the front. I had popped up to 88 pounds that year. Mind you, in kindergarten I had only weighed 33 pounds. I looked at the teacher and very seriously answered her no. She laughed. I was an extremely shy child. That was the beginning of my realization that I was *not OK*.

I remember in the second grade having the craving for canned spaghetti. Oh, so soothing for all those hurts and shows of disapproval starting to come my way. All because I was getting fat? Yes! I also loved sweet pickles. I always wanted orange juice, but could not have it that often as it cost too much. I can remember sneaking bread and going to the basement to watch TV and eat my soothing slices. I wonder to this day why mom never said anything about all the bread that was missing.

When I was about forty-five years old I suddenly recalled that a girlfriend's father had sexually abused me when I was seven years old. This was when I first began to put on weight. What was the treat afterwards? Chocolate-chip cookies and milk. I still see myself sitting at their kitchen table eating this comfort food. Oh, the pain of remembering this. To this day, chocolate-chip cookies are my best friend, next to pasta.

I never met a noodle I did not like! Pasta was and is my comfort food and binge food, even to this day. I still have to have its comfort when things really go wrong. But, at least I am now aware of the process, and understand what triggers this response of mine. For me, it has taken years to get to that point.

When I had the sexual abuse recollection, I remember before I even called my counselor, I ran to the refrigerator, got a burrito out of the freezer and threw it in the microwave and then my mouth. Oh, I felt better. I have used food for comfort. The association and comfort of how I used food was really shocking. But, I understood so much at that point of the strong lifetime relationship we (food and I) had!

Mother was a stay-at-home mom. She would bake a fresh chocolate cake every day. We would have dinner, cake and ice cream. What cake was left over went into the lunches the next day. I was always permitted to have a large piece of cake, but only three cookies. More than three was fattening. Very seldom would we have pie. Mom did not feel good about her pie crusts.

There was verbal abuse in my home, but Mom would always tell me that people "tease" those they like (love). So I learned to accept it as this is the way it is to be. Over the years, I learned to beat people at the punch line when it came to putting myself down, because if I did it first, it wouldn't hurt as badly. As I grew older, my friends finally got tired of it and kept bringing this to my attention to help me break the bad habit. Boy, was I ever taken back, as I was not aware of what I was doing.

I was in the fourth grade when I put myself on my first diet. You see, Mom did not want to help. It was the most ridiculous diet. I remember to this day, I was only having vegetable soup for lunch; 125 calories. I do not remember what I had for breakfast or dinner. I knew nothing about nutrition. Of course, I was soon hungry and Mom said basically, "I told you so." Yes. Disapproval again. I couldn't even diet right. I feel Mom always wanted me fat, so she could keep me to herself as I grew up, or tried too.

When I started junior high school it was hard for me to keep up with the others, more emotionally than physically. Junior high physical education class was not the most pleasant thing. I was always the last to be picked on teams. Oh that hurt—waiting and waiting. I was liked so much by everyone in all other ways, or so I thought, but not liked well enough to be picked first on a team.

And then having to shower with all the skinny girls was even more horrifying. I used to ask for private showers (which could be done during your time of the month), just to avoid group showering.

My real love, next to food, was music. I played clarinet in the band in junior high and was in the band, choir, and orchestra in high school. I had a hard time with the band uniforms in high school and college due to the fact my weight is in my bottom and thighs. But I managed. I started out as a music major in college, which required a lot of uniforms for various activities. Dad always said he could pick me out in the marching band because I had "such a short wheel base." My inseam is only twenty-seven inches, yet I am 5' 6" tall. Yes, I have a long torso. Something a person has totally no control over. Again, I learned to laugh it off. (What could I do about the length of my legs?) My legs were also referred to as "short, thick pile-drivers" by my family.

Moving on into high school, I found my first love. Gosh, I couldn't eat. Oh, such approval I got as I dropped a noticeable thirty pounds. What was that picture teaching me? My lunch consisted of one piece of red licorice and one instant breakfast. Lots of nutrition in that, huh? I started becoming everyone's friend. Oh that felt so good, but as we lose, we also gain. It wasn't long before I gained the weight back plus some. I always wanted to be like the rest of the girls—accepted! My best girlfriend was 4' 11" and 95 pounds soaking wet. (She and I have laughed about this for years in a very healthy manner.) My mom did not like her. She was a threat. She was going to led me astray. After all, she wore makeup, especially mascara. That was a lot of makeup in the early sixties. I was finally permitted to wear mascara and lipstick; nylons, only if I bought them. But that also required me to wear a girdle because garter belts did not come in my size. (Remember, my fullest in high school was a size 18.) This was how hard it was to be "big" in that day and age. I was also the second largest girl in my class, but I only weighed 185 pounds when I graduated from high school. Oh, how I would love to weigh that again.

As I continued to "grow," my father always referred to my bottom as "two pigs fighting in a gunny sack." How do I feel about my bottom today? Needless to say, not very good. The only way I have not had to deal with that issue, is my bottom is on the back side of me and I really don't have to look at it or deal with it, *until* I have to sit in a chair that is too small. How many of us are there? Reality check.

I never married. I can remember when I would come home from school and would tell my mother that I had a boyfriend. Her first question was always his name and, if she could not figure out what church he went to, that would be the second question. If he went to St. Mary's, then I would be told to find someone else. I never learned to judge a person for who they were and to learn from my experiences. This did not allow me to have those young fantasies that all kids (teens) need for healthy development. The boy was to be one year older than I and that was it. Period. The end. So eventually, I started finding the gay boys to hang out with. They were safe. I thought I could change them. Wrong! When I got even older, I would become infatuated with married men. Hey, they are all safe aren't they? That way I would not have to get involved with a commitment, or suffer a major hurt if it did not work out.

I went two years to a community college. I wanted very badly to get my own apartment and leave home and the bondage that had taken over my life. I was always told, "You can't do that." It did not matter what it was, "You can't do that." In my mind, I could see my apartment, me doing dishes and other household fun things. I could see myself walking to work as I would not be able to afford a car. I thought maybe I could get a job at the phone company as an operator, but again I was not the "image" for which they were looking. What image? There were no video phones in those days. Again, I was being disapproved of by someone other than the family. "Gosh, what's wrong with me? Why is everyone treating me this way?" By this time my self-esteem was close to zero.

I found my first real boyfriend in college. Someone that actually looked two times. A real date. Not just the Sadie Hawkins dance. Wow! I have a boyfriend. Well, he hurt me in a lot of ways. The first was the spring prom. He asked a skinny girl to go, not me. This was *my* boyfriend. We were inseparable. I was hurt and angry, but, nice girl that I was, I forgave him. This boyfriend will be discussed later.

I was accepted at a four-year college clear across the state. I could not wait to get away. The room and board were paid for and I could play house now, washing, ironing, caring for myself. I had my meals cooked for me. For the first time in my life I was not constipated. I learned to eat vegetables and salads. And I was walking. I remember coming home to visit on school breaks, and by the time I would go back to school, I would be so bound up it hurt. To this day, I have no problem. Was it the food or the tension from the household situations? Maybe it was both.

After maintaining a very low grade point average (all D's and F's) for several quarters, I was finally completely kicked out of school.

No wonder, I was always told I was not the student in the family and it wasn't expected of me. Another "I told you so." So why shouldn't I give up? I was slated to be a nothing, or so I perceived it. Boy, did I ever buy into that one. Mother wanted me to be a secretary, get married and have a family like she did. This was all with which she could identify. But how does a dyslexic type? Not well at all.

I had some part-time jobs while living at home and going to college. I even worked in the eating commons at school. Oh those potatoes were good out of the pan. I had a meal of potatoes while I was serving the other students, followed by dinner at the table after my shift. About three months after dropping out of school, I got a job at the county's auto license department. Six months later, I found an apartment and moved out. The actual day of moving, Mother lounged on the couch and totally ignored the whole happening. Dad helped me with everything. I was not permitted to take any furniture from the house or my bedroom, so I had to buy new things. Gosh, they were really trying to prevent the kid from leaving the house by making it harder on her financially. Maybe then she will stay.

From that point on, as I only worked six blocks from my parents' house, I was expected to come there every day for lunch. The only time I could get out of this was at Christmas. I would tell Mom to not ask questions this time of the year. This went on for two and a half years, after which I moved to a larger city. My college boyfriend lived there already. We had planned to marry. After one year in the city, I moved back to my hometown, but I was not permitted to move back in with my parents. Was this my penalty for leaving? At that particular time, I really needed the security of home, but no one was aware of the loneliness and pain that I was feeling. My boyfriend and I were soon to come to an end. I was unemployed and did get unemployment benefits, but not enough to stretch for everything I needed. Most importantly food. Since I wasn't permitted to come home, I went and got food stamps. Oh, the shame I brought on the family for doing this. I could have had money if I needed it. But I had gotten stubborn enough that I was not going to be owned by owing my parents money. I was going to do it my way. Within four months I had a good job and was off all assistance. But there was no approval from home yet. I was still made to feel incomplete.

By this time I should have been married. Why wasn't I? I was twenty-six years old. Again I was getting disapproval for this. The boyfriend went his own way and I mine. We had been dating for eight years. I took this separation as something very personal. What had I done wrong? He just walked away and never had contact with me again! I spent the next twenty years wondering where I went wrong, what could I have done differently. Needless to say, I crawled back into my protective shell and stayed there for years. Food was my friend, and boy was it. By now I had reached my all-time high of 275 pounds.

To comfort myself after this separation, I found food. I discovered that I had allergies very badly. For almost three years I gave myself shots three times a week for them. At that point the shots were for mold in the air, animals, pollens, etc. After three years I asked why I had never been tested for food allergies. I was allergic to everything tested except rye, eggs, peanuts, pure chocolate and tea. Now, you make a balanced eating program out of that. But the blessing of this came with the knowledge that beet and cane sugar along with wheat were my worst enemies. I worked very hard at cutting these out of my life. Sugar made the biggest difference at that point. I also discovered about this time that I was hypoglycemic which encouraged me even more to use sugar substitutes.

Before I made the effort to get away from my hometown, my meals were positively atrocious. My dinner day after day was a big box of macaroni and cheese followed by a quart of some kind of chocolate ice cream. (Yes! Remember the wheat and sugar allergies?) I could not understand why I felt horrible all the time.

I found myself moving away from my hometown and back to the city where I used to live. A girlfriend and I found an apartment and lived together for two years. She did most of the cooking for us, and for the first time in my life, I found out what all one could do with food. This started another one of my weight losses, just eating correctly. But after two years, we each got our own places to live. I resumed a lot of my old eating habits. While we did live together, she had grown afraid of me at times as one day I would be happy and fun, go to bed and wake up the next day so depressed and angry that I was almost nonfunctional. Without my knowing, she found an article in one of the health magazines that talked of an association between wheat and depression. Already knowing that I was wheat allergic, I eliminated wheat from my life. Boy, what a difference. Not only did my nose clear of blowing, but my attitude was 100 percent better. I actually started liking *me* for the first time in my life. I could actually feel sludge cleaning out of the intestinal area. I had almost become afraid of going to bed, as I might not be in a good mood the next day. But, I found in time that as long as I stayed away from wheat, I would be just fine.

I put myself through computer school and found excellent work after that. I also continued onto community college working toward a A.A. degree in computer operations. Here again, I had earned two "A"s and one "B." For Christmas one year I gave a copy of my grades to my parents as a gift. Then the pressure started. Every time we talked they wanted to know how the grades were doing. This put so much pressure on me, I dropped out. Again, I got the "I told you so. We knew you were trying to do too much by working and going to school." But just to prove to myself I could do it, I later started classes and when the program was dropped from the college, I had a 3.43 GPA and was on the dean's list. That proved to me that I was capable of being a good student and that I could do it.

Even though my weight had bloomed to 300 pounds, I was able to find professional jobs, even being supervisor at two different companies. I had learned to present myself as though I was a size 5 when I went to interviews.

I have tried almost every method out there to lose weight. After trying my own way, I did Weight Watchers, urine from pregnant women, along with diet pills, Overeaters Anonymous and Nutri/System. For me, none of these resulted in a permanent weight lose. If these different programs work for you, stay with them. It was after Nutri/Systems that I went to 325 pounds and I remained at that weight for ten years. I'm not saying programs such as these don't work, they just didn't work for me. Nothing "worked."

I have lost 100 pounds three times, gaining it back each time plus some. This is how I ended up where I am now. This is why I am so afraid of trying to lose again. I know I can lose, but it's the keeping it off that is hard. I know that I'm not the only woman out there that is afraid to lose. We all love the approval we get as we lose, but what if we should fail? Can we take that again?

Five years ago at my former boyfriend's funeral, I found he had chosen an alternate lifestyle which explained why there was no place for me in his life. He died of AIDS. Why couldn't he tell me so I would not have spent years waiting and wondering what was wrong with me? I am still recovering from this. But, I have learned that I am OK.

Looking at my cousin, Melonie, has shown me that with proper nutrition and exercise of some kind, it *is* possible to lose weight and maintain that loss. I have seen the pleasure this has brought her. The fun she is having for the first time in her life, shopping in the petite departments. Oh! This is so exciting to me to think my lifetime dream could be just down a short path and, done so simply, just by making a few simple lifestyle changes.

Unlike Melonie, I made my transition to health long ago and much more gradually. I did not have the huge revelation that I must make changes or I will die. About twenty years ago, I slowly began to make small changes. I started by cutting the seven-day red meat eating habit and slowly introduced chicken, turkey and fish into my meals. I have stated for years that I may be fat but at least I am healthy. That has been my motto. But now I see that I can continue to make wiser choices that can bring me closer to a long, healthy life.

As age and weight have been advancing in the later years, I began participating in a water aerobics class about one year ago. For the first time in years, I found my knees were not aching as much. I concluded that I was beginning to strengthen the ligaments and tendons that support the knees and this was really encouraging to me. Can you imagine being free of knee pain? It is wonderful. The stairs are easier to take; now I can get extra exercise both for the knees and the body as a whole. Ask me how that feels.

This time I am going to go into this with a totally different approach. I am going for a lifestyle change. I am going to have my times when I walk, bike or do water aerobics; some form of movement. I am not going to weigh daily, weekly or monthly. I will weigh when I go for my yearly Pap smear. That way I will also get a reward for weight loss and doing my exam all at once. My progress will be measured by the way my clothes, shoes, earrings, hosiery, etc. fit. I have resolved a lot of issues and I am getting a grip on life. Yes, I was always slow to mature, slow to step out. I was, and am still very shy, and will be until I become comfortable with the setting. I have permitted my shyness to protect me, and have allowed myself to be controlled by everything except what is on the inside. This is why this lifestyle change has become exciting to me.

I find it very interesting that my cousin has had many of the same issues through which to work. We have not lived in the same city since she was four years old. It has been a wonderful and delightful time getting to really know her and I admire her greatly!

Here are the statistics!

Measurements:

	Before:	After three months
Bust	51"	49½"
Waist	48¾"	48"
7" below waist	63¼"	59½"
9" below waist	61½"	59"
Upper arms	19¾"	17¾"
Thighs	35½"	32"
Calves	23⅛"	21¾"
Fat pack		
(behind the upper knee)	29"	26¼"

The Internal Combustion Engine

The Power Within

"Well, it's two weeks into my lifestyle change. Does one really withdraw from fat? By the different way I'm feeling, I would say it is possible. I was a bit constipated for a couple of days, but with increasing the complex carbos, my body is back to normal in that manner. I'm feeling more alive in just a short period of time. This makes me wonder what I will be feeling like in a month or two. I look forward to the constant change of feeling better and having the energy to do more activity."

—Jan Heaton

You have taken the first step. You are committed to getting well. Obesity is a symptom of "dis-ease." Not a disease specifically, but a lack of balance in your life. Once you recognize where your life is out of balance, you can begin to take the steps necessary to restore that balance. Once you begin to move closer to a state of balance, your body will naturally change for the better.

You experienced our own processes of identifying imbalance in previous chapters. Now it is your turn. Perhaps you think you have completed the process already. Perhaps you don't think anything is wrong with you other than heredity. The first thing you must understand is that this process never stops. You cannot take a self-test, calculate the totals and fit yourself into someone else's plan and expect to achieve what you want. We are all individuals, thank goodness. What a boring world we would live in if we were not! Life is ever changing.

You must constantly reevaluate who you are today and who you want to be tomorrow if you expect to achieve wellness and maintain it for the rest of your life. You do not live in a vacuum. Everything that happens around you, the relationships that come and go, the stresses of everyday life and even technology has an impact on your physical, emotional and spiritual health. Lifestyle change means having the skill to evaluate yourself and the willingness to make changes as often as is necessary.

You are not the same person today that you were last week or last year. If you are truly committed to wellness, the only thing that will never change is that level of commitment.

Reflect on your childhood, your earliest memories, and try to remember all of the details, good and bad, of your life to the present. Stress is not always bad. A marriage, the birth of a baby, learning something new, even taking that dream vacation is stress. Our bodies do not know the difference between good stress and bad stress. The end result is the same. Think about how you dealt with life so far. Where do you get satisfaction? What makes you feel good? To whom and what do you turn for emotional and spiritual fulfillment? How do you feel when you are not satisfied? Not emotionally and spiritually fulfilled? How do you know that you are not feeling good? What messages is your body giving you? *What is eating you?*

Our bodies tell us when something is out of balance, even if that something is not physical. We receive messages from our body in the form of hunger, fatigue, boredom, headaches, PMS, constipation or diarrhea, heartburn, acne, allergies, mood swings, depression, poor sleep, aching muscles and joints, chest pain, and the list goes on and on and on. The first thing we think is that there must be some physical ailment. We run to the doctor and are told nothing is wrong, other than the fact that we weigh too much. We are told to lose weight through exercise, starvation and deprivation. That's easier said than done! We are not given any tools that are designed to fix the problem. Instead, we are given tools that only make the problem worse. We end up feeling more depressed and ill than we were before. And the cycle continues.

Once you have identified where the imbalances are, see if there are any you can correct in the immediate future. At this point, you probably will not yet be fully aware of what's eating you, but you will be soon. Are you working more than eight or nine hours a day at your job? Is this your choice? If it is your choice, why? What satisfaction do you receive from long hours at work? Are you using long work days to avoid a bad situation at home, to avoid loneliness or to avoid socializing with other people? Do you commute long distances? Can you negotiate to work from home part of the time? Can you find a job closer to where you live? Can you move closer to your job? Can you create quality time out of your commute by listening to books on tape or your favorite music while you drive? Can you share the ride and read or work on a hobby while you are commuting?

What happens during the hours you are not at work? Do you have children who need a ride to little league, who need to get to the dentist? Is there laundry, cooking and cleaning to do? Do you have few hours at home because you are always at work? Have you scheduled one hour out of each day for yourself? If not, what can you change to find that hour? If you have the financial resources, hire a housekeeper to come in once every few weeks. Share child transportation with other parents. Involve your children and your spouse or significant other in preparing meals and maintaining the house. Caring for an elderly or ill parent? There are many community service organizations as well as private firms available to provide quality respite care or refer you to the right people who can help you.

There is nothing more important in life than taking care of yourself. If you are not well, you cannot possibly have enough of yourself left to give to others or to your job without feeling the effects physically and emotionally. You are worth one hour a day. How much is that hour worth to you? If you can put a price on it, you have not fully committed to changing your life. This may sound a bit selfish on your part at first, but soon you and those around you will admire you for having the strength and intelligence to allow time for yourself.

Review in depth your day, from the time you wake up until the time you fall asleep at night. Take a quick survey of your day. Did you eat breakfast? Did you skip lunch? Were any of your meals eaten on the run or in a car or at a fast-food restaurant? Do you remember what you had to eat today? Yesterday? How did you feel after you ate? Were you satisfied? Were you energized? Did you want to take a nap or find some dessert? Do you snack throughout the day? Were you really hungry? How did you know you were hungry? Did you eat because food was there? Someone brought goodies into the office or there was a birthday party you attended. Your best client insisted on buying you lunch at a posh Italian restaurant and you could not possibly insult the client by declining food because you were not hungry. You could not insult the hostess at the party who had worked all day to prepare a gourmet meal. You would be uncomfortable being the only person in the office not having a piece of the boss's birthday cake.

Eating for any reason other than hunger is insulting your own body. You are making choices in life that make others happy, not choices that make you feel good. If any of the above eating situations applied to you in the last few days, ask yourself, "Am I out of control?" "How do I know?" Think of a flashing red light each time you identified one of those situations. The next time you find yourself eating when you are not hungry (or not eating when you are really hungry), maybe you will see the flashing red light and regain your control. Your flashing light will disappear once you incorporate healthy changes into your lifestyle. You won't need it anymore. Then, when you are involved in a social event involving food, you will proudly decline the chocolate cake, not because you have enormous will power, but because your body has adapted to low-fat, low-sugar eating. If it gets anything but quality fuel, you will feel ill! It's easy to "just say no" when you know if you don't, you will get sick. Other people won't understand that concept. They will think highly of you because of your "will power." Let them think what they want and you enjoy the results. You will know it is not will power, but the power of your will that is resulting in achievement of your goals!

Focus your attention away from food and onto activity. Did you get some sort of physical activity today? Yesterday? Can't remember the last time you walked more than a block? When you last went to the grocery store, or if you drove your car to work, where did you park? Do you naturally tend toward the parking space closest to your destination? When you are faced with a choice between lots of stairs or a handicapped ramp, or lots of stairs and an elevator or escalator, which do you chose? If you have a store, bank, library or post office within one mile of your home or office, do you typically drive or walk when you need to visit one of these places? When was the last time you participated in the same activities that gave you enjoyment as a child? If you play golf, do you drive an electric cart or walk the course? Do you do your own house maintenance such as painting and lawn care, or do you hire it done? Do you have the other members in the family take care of these things? What do you do for fun? When was the last time you devoted an entire day to play?

While thinking of the answers to these questions, how many times did you find your activity associated with food? Isn't it amazing how whenever people get together, whenever there is a holiday, everything is focused around what time you eat? Often the activity is the food! A barbecue, a potluck, an open house or baby shower. Food is always there. A christening, a funeral, a wedding, a graduation party. When someone passes away, what is your first thought? *I should fix a casserole or something for them, they won't want to cook.* Then, you prepare the casserole, but make two so you can have one for yourself. Of course you have to taste everything as it goes in. And what about those few spoonfuls that won't fit in the baking dish, perhaps still warm from preparing the meat. "Not enough to save for lunch, and I don't want to throw good food away, so I will eat it." What about the simple act of going to the mall or the grocery store. Every mall has a food court these days. You walk in the door and smell the cinnamon rolls baking. Suddenly you're famished. You enter the grocery store and make your first turn. What's in front of you but often a sweet, older woman with a big smile on her face offering you a sample of the new flavor of ice cream. Worse yet, you see her sweating over a hot pan, preparing something with barbecue sauce and you just can't say no to this person who so much reminds you of your own mother or grandmother.

A person would be hard-pressed to think of one activity in a social setting that does not center around food or have food immediately available, unless it's a backpacking trip. You take along what food you will need for the time you are gone. There is no store down the street! And if you get hurt, or the weather turns bad, your trip is delayed and you have to ration your food supplies. Maybe we all should go backpacking once a month!

Now focus your attention on the people you interacted with today. It could be the rude bank teller, your boss who found yet another thing wrong with how you completed an assignment, your professor or school teacher who was having a bad day, the babysitter who did not show up, the doctor who kept you waiting for more than two hours. The car broke down and the tow truck driver took his own sweet time getting to you, then the mechanic was rude. You chose the shortest line at the department store, but ended up with the newest cashier. The other lines all moved faster than yours. The new desk you ordered over the Internet arrived with "some assembly required." Right, all fifty pieces of it and no hardware was included with the shipment. Then to top it all off, the washer overflowed while you were out, flooding your apartment as well as the one below. We won't mention what the call to the insurance company was like. After that mess was cleaned up, you discovered your cat shredded an entire package of toilet paper all over the floor!

Does any of this sound too familiar? A typical day? How did you deal with all of those frustrations? Were you angry at the tow truck driver because his delay caused you to miss lunch? Did you find yourself munching away? Do you remember what happened to that brownie you thought you had saved in the fridge? What were you feeling after these encounters, and what steps did you take to feel better? Did you go for a walk? Take a nap? Call a friend to tell him or her about your otherwise lousy day while sipping on coffee and scarfing down a bag of cookies?

What did you do last evening? Did you watch TV or do something with your family? Did you read a book or work on your hobby? Net-surfing anyone? How many times during that activity did you think of food, see food, or consume food? What triggered the thoughts and actions surrounding food?

If you have not yet gotten the message, think about this: The human body is dependent on water, food and oxygen for survival. These are our three most basic needs. Without any one of them, the human body dies. Do you get the same satisfaction from water and oxygen that you do from food? When you are depressed, angry, bored or in a social situation, do you crave hits of oxygen or drink gallons of water? Most likely not. So why do we treat food so differently? Food is fuel. Like gasoline for the car, or a battery for a radio, food provides the energy we need to live. Food provides the building blocks for our cells. Unlike oxygen and water, food satisfies us through taste, smell, texture and sight. Food can be experienced through all of the senses. No other life-sustaining substance satisfies us the way food does.

Food also influences your mental state. Carbohydrates, especially simple carbohydrates like pasta and sugar, give a quick blood sugar rise and resultant increase in energy. They also release a chemical in the brain that acts both as an antidepressant and a relaxant. The next time you crave chocolate or potato chips, think about how you are feeling at the time of the craving. Are you tired, depressed, angry, nervous or stressed? How do you feel after eating the chocolate? Do you feel more at ease? More tolerant? More energized? Satisfied?

We could write many chapters on the chemical effects of food, but many others have done that. Our purpose is not to give you an in-depth basic or not-so-basic chemistry or physiology lesson. Our purpose is to provide you with simple information and a common-sense approach to changing how you feel. (But just to make sure you are not disappointed, you will get a mini-biochemistry lesson in a later chapter.)

After having read this section, you may be more aware of your emotions. Try to get in the habit of ten minutes of distraction the next time you think you are hungry, or the next time you know you are *not* hungry, but crave some sort of food. Run an errand, dust the living room, start your grocery list, start a letter to a friend, do anything but sit in front of the TV. Occupy your mind. Often times, one activity will lead to another, and you may not think about food again until you stop to think about what you should do next. Really look at what activities trigger you to eat. Is it watching TV? Talking on the phone? Surfing the Internet? Putting away the groceries or preparing a complicated recipe?

Learning to differentiate hunger from the myriad other needs of your mind and body will always be one of your greatest challenges. Melonie has always had problems with blood-sugar control. She does not usually feel hungry in the same way others may. Her stomach does not make noise or get uncomfortable. When she is hungry, she gets sleepy, irritable, light-headed and shaky. She looks pale and can hardly put one foot in front of the other. When she starts to feel this way, she stops and reflects on how many hours it has been since she has eaten. If it has been three hours or more, she knows she needs something to eat. If her last meal was rather large, or contained more fat than usual, and if she hasn't had any fluids in several hours, she first drinks a glass of water. She waits ten minutes to see how she feels. If she still feels the same way, she will eat a little something. Within a few minutes, she is feeling back to her old self again. If she doesn't eat, she falls asleep and wakes up with a terrific headache. Food will ease the headache some, but it is usually after a night's sleep that the headache goes away. It's interesting to note that Melonie's mother always knew when Melonie was hungry before Melonie did. Her mother said Melonie would wilt, like a flower without water. As soon as she ate, she perked back up again, just like the flower after it has had a drink.

When Jan's blood sugar gets low, and her hunger signals kick in, she gets very quiet. She becomes lethargic and feels sleepy. Sometimes she experiences blurred vision. Like Melonie, Jan's stomach seldom growls. Give Jan a meal and within five minutes she begins to wake up and feels alert again.

It takes a lot of practice to learn what your body needs and when it needs it. No one is perfect all of the time. We catch ourselves nibbling away periodically, but the difference now is that we do catch ourselves. Stop and ask yourself, "Am I really hungry?" Most often the answer is no. Occupy your mind with something else, and balance out the indiscretion at the next meal. If you have had an especially active day, perhaps you walked two more miles or thirty minutes longer than usual, or added hand weights to the walk, then you may get hungry every two hours. You will learn if this is the case, that it is OK to eat, as long as the food is the fuel your body needs to replace electrolytes and nutrients, and build muscle.

Consciously listen to your body. Learn what it is telling you and why. This is the first step to changing your life. Never stop practicing this exercise in listening to your body signals. As soon as you start ignoring what your body is telling you, you will begin to backslide into old patterns. Food is an addiction. As with other addictions, the person who relies on food to make them feel better or to help them cope will never be "cured." The new changes you make today you will need to keep making for the rest of your life. That is why this book is really focused on lifestyle change, not diet. Dieting only makes you fat, sick, and promotes a negative self image. BodyLogic helps repair all of those years of self-destructive behavior!

Here is your first lesson in BodyLogic. Go through your house and collect all of those old diet books. Then place your scale on top of the whole stack. Walk out to the garbage can, smile and throw all of it away, and send the diet mentality in your mind with it! Free yourself of dieting. Free yourself of deprivation. Feel excitement for the journey you are about to take. Go for a short walk, then go back inside and read the next chapter!

"About four weeks into my lifestyle change, a friend asked me, 'Why are you doing this? What do you hope to gain?' My reply was this: 'I'm almost fifty years old. I want to be around for another forty years or so, and I don't want to spend that time being too sick and too big to move around. I have decided that the time is right for me to get my life in order, to make some changes that will mean something real. I'm doing this for me, for the me I am now and for the me I want to be."—Jan Heaton

Your positive self statement for today: I love myself as I am today. The love for myself is not measured by the size of my body.

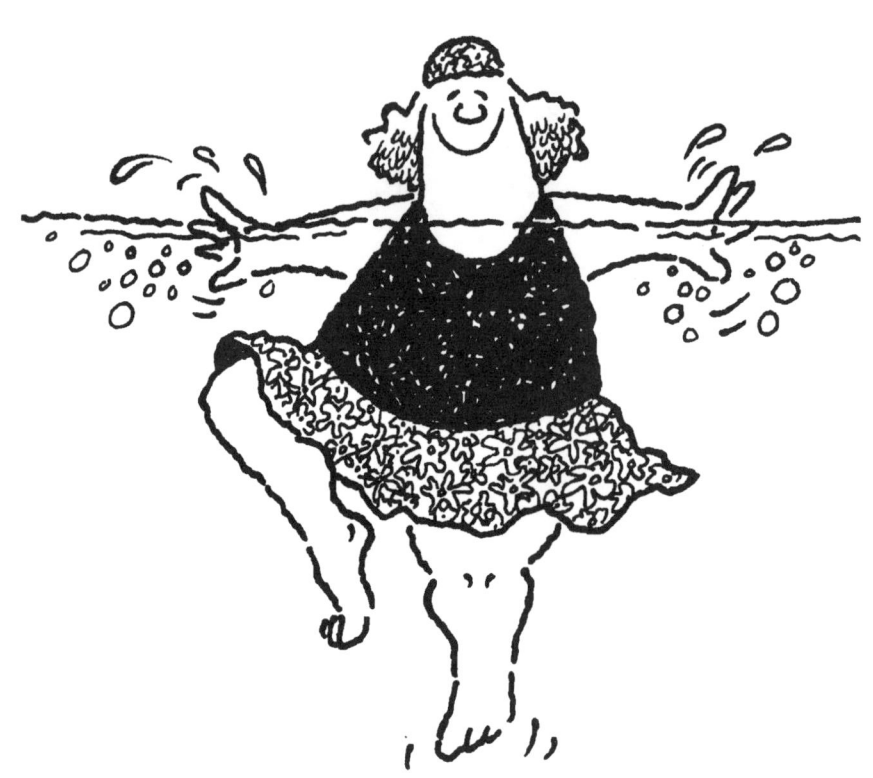

Tune-Up Time!

*Move, Baby, move! Call it what you will. If it looks like a
duck, walks like a duck, and talks like a duck, it must
be a duck—or Mel power-walking.*

*If you know what to expect, you are more likely
to try something the first time, and more likely to keep
on doing it!*

Why did we place this chapter before the one on food? The answer
again is balance. With less activity, your body needs less fuel. The
larger the body, the more fuel it needs. Activity and body weight
determine the amount of fuel you need. Just as a car burns more gas
when it covers a lot of miles, goes up numerous hills and while the
air conditioner is running full blast on a hot day, your body uses
more fuel when more physical demands are made of it. The word
"exercise" is no longer in our vocabularies. (We will use it here because you may have not reached this level of personal growth yet.)
When you reflect on the past twenty-four hours, ask yourself if you
have had an active day or an inactive day. Review your activity level
when you ask yourself if you are really hungry and factor that in as
you make your decision to eat versus engage in some other activity.

You've heard it before. Moderate physical activity increases your
metabolism. Yes, you burn more fuel (carbohydrates, protein and fat)
while you are doing a moderate activity than you do when you are
sitting. However, the real benefit comes after the activity has stopped.
This is called "after-burn," similar to the same process a jet aircraft
goes through after igniting its engines. This is the time when muscles
recover from all of the exertion. Muscle healing requires protein.
Blood sugar is depleted during moderately heavy activity. While doing the activity, your body uses the sugar it has immediately avail-

able, mainly from the last meal. When that is gone, your body relies on its fat stores for energy, to replace what it lost during exercise. Fat is broken down into glucose (simple sugar). Fat is our pantry, our emergency food supply. When we consume more than we use, the extra fuel not needed at the time is stored as fat for use later.

You likely have noticed that men lose weight much more quickly and easily than women do. Women were created to bear children. Carrying a baby for nine months requires a lot of fuel, both for the mother to deal with the extra weight of a pregnancy, and to nourish the baby. A woman's hormone cycles prepare her for childbirth. Her body naturally stores more fat in order to sustain itself during pregnancy. This is a protective mechanism, an emergency back up store of fuel. In the event enough food is not available, mother and baby will have enough fuel stored to survive. Mother Nature was right on target in this regard, at least for our early ancestors who relied on a successful hunt for their food supply. A grocery store was not available in those days.

Unfortunately, our natural processes and instincts did not change as the human race progressed. Food is now abundant for most of us, but our bodies don't realize that. Once our society became "civilized" with all of its conveniences, our bodies didn't notice. If they had, they would have said: "Oh, abundant food supply forever. No need for the food cellar anymore. Time to stop storing it up for an emergency." It is up to us to control the amount of fuel that is stored. This is most effectively accomplished by increasing activity. If you decrease fuel, your body may not have enough of the nutrients it needs to live in a healthy way. When you don't eat enough, your body senses starvation and starts storing fat. The human body requires high octane fuel twenty-four hours a day, even during sleep. It takes energy to keep muscles moving during the act of breathing. It takes energy for kidneys to function. Just as the power supply in a house does not go off when the light switch is turned off at night, neither does the body's need for energy cease when it sleeps. Anything that moves and reproduces requires fuel. Every cell, every organ, even muscle and bone are in a constant state of activity and require a constant supply of energy in order to function properly. The brighter the light, the more powerful the engine, the more energy needed. When the body does not get enough fuel, it acts like a bear, preparing itself for a long stretch without food by storing fat. It's that simple.

Physical activity increases the blood supply available to our organs. Blood carries oxygen, nutrients and water. Physical activity is to the body as a turbo engine is to a car, or as a Pentium processor is to a computer. It allows the human body to react faster and go farther. Think of the *Concord*. It keeps going for a long time and at a rapid pace because it uses high-grade fuel and only stores what it can use. Physical activity increases the size of our muscles which makes us feel stronger. Physical activity also releases chemicals in the brain that relax us, energize us and make us feel good. It strengthens the heart, and improves the function of every organ including the skin, the colon, the bones and the brain. It has been documented through scientific research that women who are more physically active have less osteoporosis as they age, fewer hip fractures, less loss of height, and no buffalo hump in their upper spine.

Like food, physical activity gives us energy, even though we use energy when we are participating in the activity. Did you know that your body needs fuel to make use of the food you give it? Physical activity impacts all of our senses like food does. When you are doing something outside, you smell the flowers, you feel the breeze in your face and the heat of the sun (or the cool of the rain here in the Northwest), you taste your sweat and you are engulfed with visual stimulation.

Do you see the connection? Physical activity is a powerful substitute for food when it comes to satisfying any need other than true hunger.

Another word we refuse to say is "workout." To a fat person who hates exercise, workout means the same thing: more structure, more regimented schedules, a forced competition with yourself to do better and better. Melonie explains it this way:

> I used to be the most inactive, anti-exercise person you would ever want to meet, next to Jan! I thought it was the exercise I hated. Wrong! It took me years to understand this one: It's not exercise you hate, it's your physical ability *to* exercise that you hate. This translates into not liking your body. How can you like your body when it hurts to move? A weak body hurts when the muscles have been stressed. A strong body also hurts when muscles are pushed beyond the limit. The difference is, weak muscles are slower to recover and hurt more when stressed than strong muscles

do. I learned to like exercise (or activity, or my hour of solitude...whatever you call it) the moment I stopped hurting so much and began to tolerate the look of my body in a pair of shorts enough to wear them in public. I really began to like it when I achieved such a state of fitness that I began to experience the high a runner often describes after a long run. No, I don't run, but I walk as fast as some joggers, and when I'm done, I am relaxed, stress free, and have this feeling of exhilaration that I cannot describe. Another benefit I noticed is the dramatic decrease in PMS symptoms as well as the pain associated with Mr. Monthly Visitor.

Here are some candid thoughts from Jan, who has been learning and using BodyLogic for several months now:

Unlike Mel, I have always had a lot of endurance. For five years I worked seven days a week. At times, those weeks would be eighty-hours long. My friends always asked, "How do you keep going? I admire your endurance." I was very regimented in my sleep, food, and extra household chores I did on a weekly basis. I had to be. I made sure I ate well, sometimes too well. I would eat four to five meals a day, not snacks, but meals! In June 1996, I dropped my forty-hour-a-week main job and decided about three months later to run my business full time. In September 1996, I decided to do something for myself. I had worked long and hard for such a long period of time, I felt it was time for me. My girlfriend and I joined a water aerobics class at the local college pool. She is 5' 10" and was 525 pounds, and myself at 5' 6" and 325 pounds, we made a real picture coming into class. It took a lot of courage for us to put bathing suits on these bodies. In one year, my friend lost 100 pounds. I did not notice the weight fall off, but I did drop a pants size just from getting the body moving.

At first there were some movements I was unable to do, as the knees were not willing, but the head was. About six weeks into the class, I was doing this one movement. I guess my eyes were popping out of my head and my friend asked if I was OK. I said, "Look! I'm doing it!" There was no pain. This was the beginning of my realizing that this is an excellent exercise program for me. To this day, I still am in water aerobics and enjoying it very much.

In the fall of 1997, I got a tune-up for my bicycle. I am ready to roll, but I'm still addressing the issue of people making fun of my fat butt and wondering where the actual bike seat stops and my backside starts. I feel like making a sign that reads: IT USED TO BE BIGGER. HONK YOUR HORN FOR SUPPORT, BUT PLEASE DON'T LAUGH. AT LEAST I'M TRYING! Can you imagine how big that sign would have to be? I really do plan on riding even in the wet Northwest fall and winter. I also have a goal of walking at least one day a week, working up to thirty minutes of that activity.

I am really determined to get this body moving and changing. I have been afraid *all* my life of allowing myself to have fun and to live. As I am almost fifty years young, I am choosing to start living! I think it will be a real adventure!

The more you move, the more fit you become. The more fit you become, the more energy you have to get through an active day. The more energy you have, the more active you will be. The more active you are, the more calories you burn. The more calories you burn, the more fuel you need! See how it all works together?

The same theory works in reverse. You see, exercise is not just about weight loss. Your body demands it to function at its peak. Think again about a car. Ever hear some people explain the difference on the wear and tear on a car between city miles and highway miles? Ever notice how much better gas mileage you get on the highway than in the city? The same concept works with the body. If your life is stop and go, stop and go, your body uses food much less efficiently than it does when it is regularly running at a higher speed. This doesn't mean you need to literally run twenty-four hours a day. Exercise increases metabolism by increasing muscle mass. An increased metabolism runs at a higher speed all day. Someone who does not exercise has a slower metabolism and runs at a lower energy level all day long.

The thin person who has been fortunate enough to be thin all of his or her life, likely engages in regular physical activity. For this lucky soul, the activity is fun. They look good in a bathing suit or sweat pants, and various body parts stay in place when they move. It seems they can eat whatever they want, but you seldom see a thin person eating constantly. Instead they are often in a constant state of movement. When not at work, their days are filled with biking, hiking, running, skiing, in-line skating, dancing or participating in some sort of competitive sport. For these people physical activity is fun. It is their social life. It is their hobby. It is what gives them the most pleasure. These are the people who are driven totally insane by being confined to the house or a hospital room. Not all thin people live like this. Melonie's mother was a perfect example. She was skinny as a rail and didn't participate in physical activity until she was forced to. She was given the choice to move or die. How much fun is that?

Being fat robs us of life's pleasures. How much fun is it to be a wallflower at the school dance? It's a lot more fun than baby-sitting on senior prom night. How much fun is strutting your 220 pounds in a swimsuit on the beach with all of those eyes staring at you and children laughing the moment you walk by? How about going water skiing when the life jacket won't buckle? How much fun is the fat child having playing softball, being called "tubby" or worse, and always being the last person selected to be on a team in gym class? How fun is it to go to purchase or rent ski's when you have to reveal your weight to a total stranger? How fun is it to go for a walk, sweat profusely, and then develop a rash where skin folds have been rubbing together? How fun is ice skating or in-line skating when your ankles are so weak that you can't hold yourself up? How much fun is riding a bike when you can't ride for five minutes without being out of breath and having your bottom hurt from the pressure of excess weight on the seat? Even riding a sled or going inner-tubing in the snow is no fun when you are so heavy that the sled or innertube won't move down the hill.

Have we pushed any buttons? Have we been there, done that, and at one time promptly refused to try any of those things ever again? You bet.

Not all fat people avoid participating in such activities. Many are not self conscious about their weight. However, they often do not appear to be having much fun in the process. They are short of breath, they sweat after two minutes of movement, they can't keep up with their kids. Their faces get this expression of being starved for oxygen, similar to the person with emphysema gasping for air. The next time you go to a park or local recreation center, observe the crowd. Compare the number of fat parents watching their children to thin parents playing with their children, enjoying the same activity.

Take a tour through your local athletic club. Look at the people in the room. You will find two types of people there. We call the first type the "Jocks and Jills." They are in competition with themselves and others to see how big their muscles can get, how much weight they can lift and how long they can work out before they collapse. These people thrive on competition, structure, regiment and enjoy showing off their bodies. The other type we call the "Got to Give Them Credits." These are people who are out of shape or in the process of getting into shape. They are either forced into the gym by their doctors because of a health problem (most often recovering from a heart attack or an injury) or they have forced themselves into the gym by being obsessed with losing weight. When you look around, how many of these people appear to be having the best time of their lives? They are sweaty. They grunt. They moan. They huff and puff. They scrunch up their faces. They stare at the TV for diversion. They count reps. They count miles. They watch every minute. We don't call that fun. To each his own. Needless to say, we are not members of a gym.

Melonie will share with you her own personal experience with exercise. She will be admitting many mistakes. We all have lessons to learn. If her experience will help you to have a pleasurable lifestyle change, this book has fulfilled every expectation we had for writing it. You are more likely to repeat an activity if you enjoy it. Here are some candid accounts from Melonie's lifestyle-change process:

My lifestyle change was motivated by a deep desire to feel good. I did not embark on this new path with the goal of losing weight or to become a body builder or a marathon runner. I just wanted to make it through an entire day like "normal" people. Normal people do not sleep fourteen hours out of every twenty-four. Normal people do not decline invitations because they are unable to keep up with their friends, no matter what the activity is. When dining in a restaurant, my friends who ordered the same meal as I always had larger portions on their plates. The waitress would always say, "We ran out of french fries. I'll bring you more when they are ready." She never did. My lifestyle change was not motivated by wanting to *be* normal. What is normal anyway? All I wanted was to feel better tomorrow than I did today. After all of my reading, I decided increasing my physical activity was worth a try. If I didn't give it a chance, how would I know if it would help me feel better?

I have always been the type of person who enjoys immediate satisfaction from a job well done. If my first attempt at something wasn't perfect, I would give it two more tries. If it still wasn't perfect, or if I didn't get what I wanted after three tries, I would give up and find something else to go after. In addition, I never started anything at the beginning. When I learned to cook, I chose a complex recipe rather than a simple one. When I taught myself to do counted cross stitch, I started on the tiniest count fabric. When I decided to experiment with wallpaper, I chose to do an entire bathroom rather than one wall. There have been few things in my life I have devoted a lot of time and effort to. Nursing school was one. Starting and running two businesses is another. I think the only other thing I ever stuck with was playing the clarinet. Eventually, I succeeded at all of these endeavors. The secret here is that I enjoyed them, and I wanted them almost more than life itself.

Unfortunately, when it came to getting my body moving, I did not think of the long-term payoff. I was willing to give it a try for a while, and if it didn't "fix me," I would find something else to try. This revelation came on my thirty-fourth birthday, the month was March. My goal was to be *well* (not *thin*) by the end of the year. So I started to, here it comes, "work out." "Exercise." Mistake number one. By categorizing physical activity in this way, I immediately developed the attitude that this was something I had to do, every day, exactly on the schedule described in the magazine, the book, or on the video tape. I chose activities that I could do in the privacy of my own home, away from judgmental eyes and on my own schedule. I tried the aerobics and stair-stepper videos. I couldn't keep up with the beginner level. I gave up on those activities, and decided to start from square one.

Step one was walking. I poured myself into sweatpants and a sweatshirt, an old pair of tennis shoes, bought a watch with a second hand on it so I could check my pulse, and off I went. I will never forget day one. I think I made it all of five minutes. My pulse was racing. My legs cried out in pain. I was short of breath and sweating profusely. I was very disappointed in myself because the book said I should start with fifteen minutes a day. Instead of giving up, I threw away the book, and found a more sensible one.

It said to start out at a level of intensity that is comfortable for you, and gradually increase your time, distance and pace. This I could do. Someone gave me permission to be me! Day two was no better. I had spent the night with leg cramps and didn't sleep at all. When I got up my back hurt and I was exhausted. I did not walk that day, but I did walk on day three. It was much the same as day one, but I survived. By the end of week number two, I had increased my walking time to fifteen minutes. I learned to start slow and pace myself, rather than trying to fit into someone else's plan of "four miles per hour, one hour a day, every day." By week number three, I began to feel different. I noticed the leg pain was gone. I was sleeping better. I was able to go without my afternoon nap on the days I exercised.

Could it be that I chose to give up my nap to fit in a walk? Was my poor physical condition only part of the reason I couldn't stay awake in the afternoon? I didn't think too much about it at the time. I was just happy to stay awake all afternoon. I didn't care why.

The weeks passed slowly. After eight weeks, I noticed my clothes had started to fit a little differently. Oh no, mistake number two. I got on the scale. (Note: Please learn from Melonie's mistakes in this regard. It is much easier to prevent scale obsession than it is to cure it! Melonie continues to struggle with this on a daily basis, but the scale does not get used as frequently as it did before.) I had lost five pounds. I had more energy. I was beginning to sense strength in my legs that I had not felt before. I was elated. I thought, this exercise stuff works. I wonder if changing my diet would move things along any faster, or have any impact on the way I felt? Stepping on that scale started two years of pure obsession with my weight. I quickly forgot about my goal of just wanting to feel better. I would get on that scale three times a day. Happy when the weight went down, and devastated when it went up. When the weight went up, I worked out harder, often beyond my limits.

Over the next year, I was ever faithful to my workouts. If I didn't sweat, I didn't think I had exercised to my full potential. For the first year, my only physical activity was walking. I really got into it. I bought a decent pair of shoes, exercise clothes that were comfortable and that made me feel good to wear, a Walkman and workout music. I found some wonderful tapes, with the beat matching a certain pace. My first tape was for "beginners." It was three miles per hour for thirty minutes. I began this tape about month number three, not being able to finish the entire tape at first. I ignored the "for beginners" classification and kept on moving. Mistake number three. I soon found myself engaging in my own private competition. I would push harder and harder, to increase my time, distance and pace. Again I went overboard. The muscle pains came back. I sweat a lot. I would walk until I almost collapsed. Some days I wondered if I would ever make it back home. I always did. I had attempted to advance myself way too fast. In two short months, I was pushing myself to 3.6 mph. And I kept going.

The beginning of month six, on Labor Day weekend, the anniversary of my mother's death, I was starting to get bored with my workouts. I had myself on a very structured schedule, allowing myself to miss only one day a week, and often putting myself down if I missed that one day. What I didn't learn from the books—mistake number four—is that muscles need time to recover. If you are over thirty, and/or your body is complaining, you should wait twenty-four hours between the same kind of exercise sessions, and alternate activities on a daily basis. If you are under thirty, and you are not experiencing discomfort, repeating the same exercise daily is fine, as long as you give yourself those twenty-four hours of recovery time. On weekends and holidays, I would walk twice a day, morning and night, to make up for that one day I missed earlier in the week. I found myself suddenly lacking in energy, unable to walk the same distance I had the week before. I was bored, I was tired, and I hated the fact that for all my effort, and all those missed "Oprah" episodes, I was backsliding. I was gaining weight.

I needed diversion. I bought a mountain bike. I started slow for once, but again advanced too quickly. By the time the rains came in late October, I had attempted a twenty-mile ride, again, almost not able to make it home. My legs hurt. I was exhausted. Mistake number five: I did not learn from mistake number three (being in a competition with myself and moving beyond my body's capability). I bought a manual treadmill and set it up in my bedroom. I figured I could walk indoors that way, now that the days were shorter and very wet. Mistake number six. I bought cheap exercise equipment that I had not tried out first. It had belonged to a friend and had been sitting in her garage for two years. Needless to say, it would have taken a tractor to get that belt to move. I returned the favor and sold it to another friend. It's still folded up in her closet! I got smarter. I bought an electric treadmill, one I had tried out first. It had all the bells and whistles, and to be honest with you, was the best investment I ever made.

During the winter, I walked five days a week, using the other two days for muscle recovery. I also started lifting weights on those off days. The boredom continued, but I learned to plan treadmill time during "Oprah" or some other TV program I enjoyed. The bike sat in the garage during the winter, and the spring. It made an appearance in late summer. I went riding a few times but was frightened to be out on the busy streets. Mistake number seven. I should have researched safe biking trails and planned fun scenic trips during the summer. By the time I made that discovery, summer was gone. The rains came again, and I found myself staring at that treadmill with daggers in my eyes. By this time, one and a half years into my lifestyle change, I had learned that if I don't do some activity most days of the week, whether it be walking or biking, if I do not exert myself regularly, I quickly fall back into the same old patterns. Fatigue sets in. I ache. I get headaches. I don't sleep well. I start munching indiscriminately, or I start starving myself because the scale won't budge or moves in the wrong direction. I become irritable. I quickly fall into an "I don't care" attitude.

Some days it takes every bit of motivation I can muster, but I get off my backside and move. Within minutes of dragging myself onto the treadmill, the bike, or the walking path, I begin to feel better. I remind myself that walking increases the enzymes in my muscles that help burn fuel for energy. This is the one hour in my day free of interruptions, demands, phones, the pager and sitting in traffic. This is my time to relax, recharge, and reflect. This is when I do my best thinking. My head clears. I notice what a beautiful city I live in. What keeps me going now is the fear of feeling like I did several years ago. It's much easier to maintain my current level of fitness and health than it was to achieve it in the first place. I never want to re-live those first eight weeks of agony. But

I notice one and one-half years later, the feeling that something is still missing. For the next six months, I continued to engage in physical activity four or five times a week. Then one day while riding my bike, two years and three months later, that I realized I was really enjoying my ride. In fact, I woke up that morning and couldn't wait to hit the bike trail. I couldn't get dressed fast enough. It was early morning. All of the spring flowers were in bloom. The waterway that runs next to the trail was full of baby ducks and geese. Not a two-footed creature was on the path, nor a two-wheeled contraption, other than mine. The sounds of the birds singing their early morning songs. The smell of the flowers. The feel of the crisp breeze in my face. The taste of the fog in the air that day. There were two hot-air balloons following the waterway, floating so low I could hear the "hiss" of the air.

For the first time in my life, I felt alive. The next day, I awoke with the same desire I had the day before. I chose a walk down my favorite walking path, away from the city streets. I experienced all of the same sensations I had the prior day. This time I was treated to a family of wild rabbits out gathering their morning meal. I was totally relaxed and at peace with my life. That is the time when I had, unconsciously, released myself from workouts and exercise, and began to participate in physical activities that I enjoyed. It was no longer a struggle to get motivated. I had incorporated fun activities into my lifestyle. Moving my body became fun because my body was strong. I will never work out or exercise again. From now on, I will have fun on a regular basis. Now, fun is seeing if I can ever become a racewalker and compete. Yes, I know that sounds like some of that competitive spirit mentioned before, but the difference is this is fun and I don't put myself down if I don't increase my speed or distance every few months.

You know what fun is? It's walking twelve-minute miles with hand weights, singing to my boogie tunes, passing up many joggers on the trail. Fun is having people look and smile at me, and stop me to ask how I get my short legs to go so fast! Fun is having people not even notice me because I no longer have all of the flab that used to move harder and faster than I did. That really drew attention. I now schedule "Fun Breaks" into my day. That may sound somewhat silly, but each person incorporates new learning into their daily life in a different way. But you must also remember, just like food, alcohol, drugs or any other addiction, exercise can be addictive too, and it is easy to backslide into that personal competitiveness that causes you to move at a level beyond your limits.

After a few years, you get to know your body very, very well, and those extreme sessions become fewer and fewer. Progression becomes much more natural. Speed and endurance are increased because your fitness level has increased, and the old speed in the old time are too easy. You will know when the time is right to advance a level. It doesn't matter how you do it, or what you call it, as long as you live it and not just practice it.

No chapter on exercise would be complete without a few words of caution. 1) If you have any medical problems for which you are under a doctor's care, please see your doctor before you begin any exercise program. 2) If you are very out of shape, get out of breath just walking a few feet, are over thirty-five or have a history of heart or respiratory disease in your family, see your doctor first before starting your program. While walking is probably the most convenient and inexpensive exercise for most anyone, water aerobics, swimming or using a bike might be more appropriate for you depending on your overall health status and bodyweight. Most of all make it fun! Why shouldn't you try martial arts, volleyball, tennis, ice skating or roller skating. Take up golf. Try horseback riding. Play Frisbee with the kids or the dog. Winter time? How about snowshoeing? Exercise does not have to be boring or competitive. Do whatever you like, as long as it gets you moving and keeps you moving for a period of time that you can physically tolerate, even if it's five minutes. Start slow and work toward your goal. You will be amazed at how fast you will progress, and how much fun you can have during the process!

You likely have heard many things regarding the best time of day to exercise. Listen to your body. If you are a morning person, plan your activity for first thing in the morning. If you are a night person, you may feel more energetic in the afternoon or evening. Experiment. Find out what time of day feels best and fits best into your schedule. Many overfat people tend to have a slower metabolism in the morning, so if you can plan your activity for the morning hours, you may see more benefit in a shorter amount of time. Just get out there and do it, no matter what time it is. Schedule your activity into your day like you would anything else and stick to that schedule. Be consistent with the time of day. Mel plans her activity break first thing in the morning, right after breakfast. This way, it is the first thing that gets done. Mel finds if she procrastinates, and does not stick to her routine, she will find many other things to get wrapped up in during the day and that activity break will never happen!

There are mixed opinions regarding whether or not you should eat before you exercise. It really depends on how your body uses its fuel. Some people get nauseated if they exercise right after a big meal. That's because they move their body at a high intensity and for a long period of time. For most of you just starting out, you could probably go for your walk or whatever within thirty minutes after a meal without feeling any discomfort. You must take into account any health problems you may have. Melonie gives an example:

I am hypoglycemic and find I need good food within a couple of hours of my fun break or I literally run out of gas in the middle of my session. My body needs slow-burning, quality fuel (complex carbo-hydrates) to tolerate the intensity at which I move. You will need to experiment to find out how your meal times and exercise sessions are best planned. Listen to your body and give it what it needs!

You have probably heard about target heart rate, not allowing your heart rate to get too fast during exercise. You may find this method too complicated and cumbersome. It seems self-defeating to be moving at a comfortable pace, breathing just hard enough to speak one average sentence at a time, only to have to stop to check your pulse. We are not saying the target heart rate method is not a good idea to use. You need to make a personal decision about this, and discuss it with your doctor. You may need to have a treadmill electro-cardiogram in order to know what a safe pace is for you. Just don't move so hard that you are sucking wind and feel like you are going to die. You should be at a rate that you are moving as fast as you can while being comfortable doing it, as far as breathing goes.

In the beginning, parts of your body will scream out in pain. Think of it like this: "My muscles are waking up after a deep sleep. They are sustaining some trauma, but the healing will make them stronger than before. Within four to eight weeks, this moving thing will be much more comfortable." If during or after physical activity you experience severe pain anywhere, stop the activity and see and your doctor. You may have injured yourself. In time, you will learn what is normal muscle fatigue and what is true injury.

Most aerobic exercise (that which keeps you breathing more than normal for an extended period of time) utilizes the lower body. Don't forget to pay attention to your upper body by doing a few simple weight lifting or other strengthening exercises two or three times a week. No special equipment is necessarily required. Just remember wherever you build muscle, you have more calorie burning tissue. Muscle bulk also smooths and tones, so you look firmer. Muscle will use energy whether or not you are engaging in physical activity. You don't have to "bulk up" to get the benefit.

It is essential, no matter what activity you participate in, to warm up before and cool down after. Warm-up is done by participating in your usual activity at a very slow pace, gradually increasing your speed over ten to fifteen minutes until you reach the maximum of your comfort zone. During this time, your muscles become warm and limber. When you have completed your session, cool down in the reverse manner of the warm-up, gradually decreasing intensity until your breathing returns to normal. Warm up and cool down should take about the same amount of time. Then, you must gently stretch out the muscles you have used. Stretching relaxes the muscles, and helps to prevent pain and stiffness later. It also helps make the next session a bit easier. Without stretching, the muscles go into spasm, contract and tighten. Tight muscles hurt! Stretched muscles improve flexibility and performance. Never stretch to the point of pain, but hold each stretch for thirty to forty-five seconds. *Never* stretch a cold muscle. This can cause injury and never feels very good. Stretching prior to warm-up is not recommended.

Once you begin to get stronger, you will need to tone those abdominal muscles as well. Walking and cycling and various other forms of lower body movement will strengthen the abs to some degree. All of the abdominal crunches in the world will not flatten your stomach if it is overfat. But they will increase strength and tone, and make you feel stronger and look firmer. A flat stomach is probably an unachievable goal for most of us. Thank goodness there are undergarments to give us (or take away) what nature forgot! Perfection is not the goal. Health and feeling good is.

Finally, replenish the fluids you have lost during exercise. Melonie has a fanny pack with a water bottle on it and takes some fluid every mile or so, maybe half a cup. Drinking too much during exercise can cause nausea. Dehydration decreases your performance. It can cause fatigue and muscle pains. Again, it's about balance. After your session, drink a tall glass of water.

Sports drinks seem to be making a huge debut at the grocery store these days. Sports drinks contain sugar in addition to salt and potassium. They are designed to replace nutrients and fluids lost during exercise. Sports drinks are not necessary if your exercise time is less than an hour. Some authorities say less than two hours. This is individual. When Melonie exercises for more than an hour but less than two hours, she feels much better afterward if she drinks a small amount of sports drink. For those exercising at low intensity or for a short duration of time, these drinks probably will do nothing for you except add empty calories. Keep in mind that sports drinks were originally designed for the athlete, the marathon runner. A thirty-minute walk at a moderate pace hardly qualifies as a marathon, though it may seem like it to you right now!

After moving your body, eat a light complex carbohydrate snack such as a small piece of fruit, just to help your body recover and prevent it from thinking it is starving. Heavy people tend to get quite hungry after exercise. This is the body's self-preservation mechanism kicking in. It wants to replace the carbohydrate and fat stores it lost during the activity. Keep in mind that the body needs to move for more than twenty minutes before it starts burning fat for fuel. After exercise, your body's metabolism will be functioning at a higher rate for several hours, so it will easily burn off a small carbohydrate snack rather than storing it as fat. The trick with the light snack is to give your body the carbohydrates it needs, but not to give it any fat. We will discuss the role of carbohydrates, proteins and fats in a later chapter.

Words for the wise: Breathe, motivate and decorate! Don't forget to breathe deeply and rhythmically while engaging in physical activity. Oxygen is what makes fat burn. Oxygen helps to keep muscles from screaming out in pain because they are not getting enough air. Filling your lungs with oxygen during activity will help you de-stress, and feel much more relaxed when you are finished.

"People always ask me how I keep motivated. My motivation comes from feeling great most every day. Sure, I have days where I feel a bit sluggish, everyone does, but those are a rarity rather than the norm like they used to be," Melonie says.

We discussed before how it is not a good idea to get into a competition with yourself when engaging in physical activity. We want to clarify that point. Being too competitive will cause you to move beyond your physical capacity, causing pain and injuries. However, a little bit of competitive drive keeps you moving forward, advancing in your speed and distance. For example, if you walk to a 3 mph tape, think about how much more fun it will be when you get to pick up the beat a bit at 3.5 mph! *Don't* strive for 5 mph when you are at 3 mph.

One small step at a time. One day at a time. Allow your body to get totally bored with your current level of activity. That's when you will know it is time to advance a step. What we mean by the body getting bored is, you will notice you are not in your zone. You are not breathing hard. You may not even break a sweat. That's your body saying, "Hey, I'm more fit. Let's crank it up a notch!"

Decorate your body and you will literally feel better while moving. It's more than just how you look. Of course, moving in something that looks good and is comfortable will make it more likely that you will stick with the program. Shopping is a reward for sticking with your fun breaks for so long that all the elasticity is gone in your clothes. But there is an even more important reason to have quality clothing when you move: Reduce pain and discomfort. If your activity program involves any type of an activity, that is using your legs while weight bearing and moving (walking, jogging, running, doing aerobics, jumping rope, using the trampoline or ski machine—you get the picture), *you must first and foremost invest in a good pair of shoes* that are appropriate for the activity you are doing. Don't trust the local discount store. Take all that money you have been spending on junk food and put it into one good pair of athletic shoes. Wear your old shoes and go into an athletic supply store. We prefer those catering only to women! Talk with the salesperson about what kind of activity you plan on doing. Look at your shoes for the wear pattern and have the clerk do the same. If you have high arches it is likely that your foot rotates inward when you walk. You can tell if your foot lands in any manner except flat and straight by looking to see where the bottoms of your shoes are most worn. A foot rotating in or out will significantly result in more pain and muscle fatigue when you move. Get a good quality shoe with some flex in the sole, and good arch supports. Plan on spending no less than $75 unless you find an outrageous bargain. If you stick with your program, budget to have a new pair of shoes every three to six months, or every three hundred miles, depending on how much activity you do.

How do you know when it's time for a new pair of shoes? Listen to your body, don't look at the shoes. Melonie has at least six pair of walking shoes lying around her house in various states of wear. Other than those worn at the beach, most look pretty good when cleaned up, almost new! The soles don't look worn very much. But guess what? It's what you *can't* see that counts. In every one of those pairs, the inner support is gone. The cush has gone south. Wearing worn out shoes is like walking in bare feet. You don't need to look at the calendar to know when you need a new pair of shoes. *Listen to your body and here's what it says:*

- Leg pain, most everywhere, especially the fronts and backs of the thighs and calves (including shin splints).
- Hip pain.
- Ankle pain.
- Heel pain.
- Knee pain.
- Low back pain.
- Decreased stamina and/or inability to advance a level in the usual amount of time.
- Aching or painful feet.
- Morning stiffness and pain.
- Limping in pain all day long.
- Even mid-back pain, shoulder pain and neck pain can be caused from a poor gait and poorly fitting shoes.

OK. So how do you know these symptoms are from shoes and not overdoing it from trying to advance too quickly? First, do some thinking. Have you had a period of time without pain while being active? (Keep in mind you will hurt for the first six to eight weeks of any new program, but good shoes will help that.) If yes, take a day off, keep your legs up when you can, and take three or four doses of an over-the-counter pain reliever. (Check with your doctor first.) If one muscle hurts more than the others, you might want to ice it for twenty minutes several times during the day, waiting a couple of hours between each icing. You will probably wake up the next morning stiff and sore, but feel a bit better. (If your pain is severe, call your doctor.)

When it's time for your activity break, put on those shoes and go for it as usual. You may want to decrease the intensity if you had advanced your level and noticed the onset of discomfort at the same time. If it's overactivity, you will hurt, but not as bad as the day before. If it's shoes, your pain will be the same or worse during this next session. Melonie says, "I notice a gradual increase in pain over a week or so until it gets to the point where I can hardly walk my route at all. My muscles cramp up and my legs scream out." Check the calendar or the check book (or the credit card statements) to see when you made your last shoe purchase. Try to estimate how many miles those shoes have on them. Keep in mind a heavier person may not get the same wear out of a pair of shoes as a lighter person. A lot depends on how your feet land and the quality of the shoes, in addition to the intensity of movement and the type of terrain on which you move.

If your pain continues despite the off day and decrease in intensity, and you can't remember the last time you purchased shoes, go get new ones. Wear your old ones when shopping and repeat the same discussion you had with the salesperson last time. Likely, your activity level has increased, or your preference in activity has changed. Technology changes faster than you replace your shoes. Wear those new shoes the next day you do your activity. If the problem was your shoes, your legs will immediately feel better, your feet should feel like they are walking on clouds, and the closer you get to the end of your session, the better your legs will feel. If you are still in serious discomfort, you may have an injury worth seeing a doctor for, or, you may have purchased the wrong pair of shoes. Take them back. Also, if you are very large and/or notice very significant wear patterns on one part of your shoe more than the other, or if you routinely experience any of the symptoms mentioned previously, you should probably see a podiatrist who specializes in sports medicine. You may need to be fitted with a special orthotic to correct gait problems, or there may be other issues the doctor can address that will increase your comfort. *Do not* buy so-called orthotics in the store or from a catalog. There is a difference between "orthotics" and "inserts." Don't buy anything to put in your shoe that will change how your foot lands on the pavement (and some inserts will do that) without talking to a podiatrist first. You may cause more problems than you already have. Much of this may seem like trial and error. It is. In time, you learn to recognize what messages your body is giving you.

Finally, the type of clothing you wear is just as important as shoes. Get a good supporting sports bra if you can find one, or buy a couple extra bras for your activity breaks. (See chapter on bras.) Choose tops that breathe. Lightweight cotton is always good. We like just a man's T-shirt. We like them baggy. Baggy is comfortable, baggy breathes, and baggy hides a multitude of things! For bottoms, choose cotton panties. For outerwear, go back to the athletic store and find shorts or longer bottoms that are made to slightly compress you. They come in several weights so you will be comfortable in every season. What a difference they make. The fabric breathes but it keeps your muscles warm. Warm muscles are more limber and less painful. The support is like the wonderful relief similar to what you get from a good pair of support hose. Finally, what supports you will compress you. What compresses you makes you look thinner and jiggle less. All around, this is the best eighteen dollars you will ever spend for a pair of shorts. Watch for sales. Don't forget the feet once again. Invest in good socks that provide some cushion, but that whisk away moisture. These will keep your feet cool, comfortable, and prevent athlete's foot and other skin infections. Don't forget a sweatband and a hat if you are so inclined. If you cannot find exercise clothing in your size at a local specialty shop, there are mail-order options available or you may have to make them yourself or have them specially made for you. Specialty shops will be listed in your local telephone directory or will have advertisements in women's magazines.

The BodyLogic Top Ten List

Let's get blunt for a moment. We know all of the excuses for not exercising. We have a valid response for most every one of them, so from here on out, no more excuses:

The top ten reasons why I cannot exercise:

1. *I don't have time.* Make the time. Schedule your activity session just like you do anything else. There are enough hours in the day, more

than enough. You would be amazed at how many lost minutes you can capture from one twenty-four-hour period. Set your alarm one hour earlier in the morning, and go to bed one hour earlier the night before. Use that first hour in the day to take time to care for yourself. This is the one hour in the day that is totally yours, free from interruptions, telephones, the kids, the pager, the cell phone. If you plan your activity breaks for first thing in the morning, nothing will get in the way of them. When finished, you have the entire rest of the day to deal with life's headaches.

2. *I can't find shoes that fit.* You can if you are creative. If you have a computer, you can find many stores that offer odd sizes by searching the Internet using the category of "athletic shoes." Mel buys her shoes this way quite often and has never been disappointed. Outlet malls are another great place to find odd-sized shoes. When just starting out, you don't need the most expensive pair you can find, just something that is comfortable and gives you good support. If you are a woman with large feet, look at men's shoes. If they are too wide, wear extra thick socks or an extra pair of socks and lace those suckers up tight!

3. *I'm too embarrassed. People will make fun of me.* Join a class like Jan did, where there are other people of similar size and shape. Find things you can do in the privacy of your own home, whether it be riding an exercise bike, using exercise videos, or rent or buy a treadmill if you can afford it. Try a mini-trampoline, a rowing machine, one of those newfangled exercise rider contraptions. Find a walking path off the street and if you can, plan your activity break for a time that the majority of other people are not out. Often times, you will find people just like you out on those trails, and not just during off-peak times either! The biggest source of embarrassment is inside of your own head. You have to develop a positive attitude. You have made one of the most important decisions in your life, the decision to get well. Nothing, but nothing should get in the way of that. Each day as you begin your activity break, say out loud to yourself, "I don't care what others think or say. I'm doing this for me. If they are so small (mentally) that they must make fun of me, then they are to be pitied. I am a bigger and stronger person than they for making a commitment to myself."

4. *I can't find clothes that fit.* Read the chapters "From Clunker to Classic" and "Headlights." Go to a discount store and shop in the

men's department. Go to a big-and-tall men's store and pretend you are shopping for someone else if you have to. You don't have to be a fashion model. Just be comfortable. As time goes on, finding clothes that fit will be much easier, and an experience you will look forward to.

5. *My feet hurt. I have heel spurs, bunions or corns, plantar fascitis, high arches, etc.* There are many cushions on the market, available in your local variety or drug store, designed just for cushioning places on the feet that need cushioning. There is a great product out there called Sports Tape. It is similar in feel to the double-sticky picture-hanging tape you use on walls. It is about one-half inch or so thick, and padded, just slightly sticky on one side. This stuff is great to put over blisters or any spot that tends to be rubbed by shoes. It will not tear the skin when you peel it off, and it holds up under wet conditions! Lambswool and moleskin also provide nice protection. If your feet cause you that much pain, then likely you are in pain at times other than during exercise. If that is the case, see a podiatrist!

6. *I'm so big that the seat on the bike slips down when I get on it. I can't seem to get the screw tight enough!* One of Mel's favorite toys is her power drill, the supercharged turbo model of course! Adjust the seat where it needs to be. Get out your drill, and drill a large hole (the width of a bolt) through the bike frame and the support rod. Insert the bolt through the hole and that support rod won't go anywhere. (Thank you, Ben Gleason, for your helpful hint!) If you are not into drills, and prefer to let someone else deal with such things, try this: put the seat in the lowest possible position, so that the rod is resting on the bottom support of the bike. Measure the length. Readjust the seat to where it should be for comfort. Figure out the total length of those two distances, go to a home improvement center, and find a metal rod of the same diameter as the one on your bike. Have the sales person cut the rod to length. Take it home, replace the old one with the new, reattach the seat, and you are ready to roll. The rod won't slide down because it's already sitting in there as far as it will go!

7. *I want to walk outside, but I don't feel safe.* Find a friend or neighbor who owns a dog, and offer to take it for a walk a few times a week. You might be keeping your friends from getting their activity, but you will feel safer, and you will have a companion to join

you. Many animal shelters welcome volunteers to walk the dogs. Start your own dog-walking business on the side. Kill three birds with one stone. Feel safe, get your activity, and make a few bucks extra to spend on some new shoes. If the dog-walking thing is not possible, place an ad in the paper for a "walking buddy." There are many groups out there who walk together several times a week. There is safety in numbers. These groups are not all that hard to find. Your local parks and recreation department would be a great place to start.

8. *I hate to exercise. I hate to sweat. I hate how it makes me feel.* Re-read this chapter! The more you do, the better it feels, and the more you will look forward to it. Have you truly made a commitment to change? Have you made a promise to yourself that is so sacred, so special, so important that you could never break it? If not, then you are not yet ready to change your lifestyle. Re-read the first four chapters of the book. Reevaluate your life. Identify what things must be in place in order for you to be ready to make the commitment. The only person you hurt by saying you will do something that you have no intention of doing is yourself!

9. *My knees hurt. My back hurts. I'm just too big!* You need non-impact activities like water aerobics, swimming, or riding an exercise bike. Do these kinds of activities first, to strengthen your muscles and start the fat burning process. As you get stronger, and the fat starts to leave your body, you will have less pain and will be more comfortable moving on to some low impact activities like walking.

10. *I am AFRAID to FAIL!* Let's look to the past to find the road to the future:

"We are all failures—at least, all the best of us are."
—*J.M. Barrie,* Rectorial Address, *3 May 1922, St. Andrew's University, Scotland.*

"Failure after long perseverance is much grander than never to have a striving good enough to be called a failure."
—*George Eliot, in* Middlemarch, *bk.2, ch. 22 (1871-72)*

"When we can begin to take our failures nonseriously, it means we are ceasing to be afraid of them. It is of immense importance to learn to laugh at ourselves."
—*Katherine Mansfield,* The Journal of Katherine Mansfield *(1927), October 1922 entry.*

"All animals, except man, know that the principal business of life is to enjoy it."—*Samuel Butler,* The Way of All Flesh, *Ch. 19 (1903)*

"It is better to be fat, and as healthy as possible, than to be skinny and sick. It is an insult to yourself to be both fat and sick if you can do something about it."—*Melonie Heaton, RN and Jan Heaton,* BodyLogic *(1997)*

We hope this chapter has given you a different view of what exercise can do not only for your body, but for your spirit. Get to know your body and listen to what it says! Have fun while moving. Learn to love your body and you will start to love moving it around! You must grow on the inside before you can shrink the outside. Grow muscles, grow heart function, grow respiratory capacity, gain control over blood sugar and increase the mileage you get out of your fuel. But most importantly, grow your inner self. Find the real you, and the rest will follow naturally. That's BodyLogic.

> ***Your positive self statement for today: In the words of Abraham Lincoln, "I'm a slow walker, but I never walk back."***

Fuel for Thought

*Food: A substance (especially solid) taken into the body
of an animal or plant to maintain its life.*
The Oxford Dictionary

It's that simple. You eat, you live. You starve, you die. We mentioned this briefly in the last chapter. Every living thing must eat in order to survive.

Unfortunately, in many cases, our role models have taught us just the opposite. We have been taught that food is pleasure, and that women, in particular, are not worthy of such pleasure. Our culture has evolved with the mind-set that women should eat like "birds." We must be dainty. To eat to our fill is not ladylike.

"For much of the female half of the world, food is the first signal of our inferiority. It lets us know that our own families may consider female bodies to be less deserving, less needy, less valuable."—Gloria Steinem. *Outrageous Acts and Everyday Rebellions,* 1983. (Quoted by permission.)

We, as women today, need to be role models for the women of tomorrow. It is up to us to change this perception about food. All food is not created equal. We promise you that no attempts will be made to try to force you to acquire our eating habits. Your culture, health beliefs and needs, religious beliefs, your food preferences and all of your life experiences have created the special individual that you are. We don't want to change those things that make you unique. However, perhaps we can teach you ways to make healthier food choices, while continuing to eat those foods that you love. A little creativity and a lot of technology have given our generation so many more choices in what we eat than our parents had. Many are for the better. Many may actually be worse. We are not anti-artificial anything. We are not vegetarians. We love peanut butter and chocolate and eat them whenever we want. You heard it before, but here it is again. It all has to do with balance. Give your body what it needs, when it needs it, and your body will take care of the rest. That's BodyLogic!

It's been one month now since I started BodyLogic. I just took my first measurements and I have lost ten inches! I can't believe it! This makes me feel good! Also, I have had to remember to *eat*, to recognize *hunger*. This is a totally different approach to what has previously been programmed into my mind, Jan says.

Here is the recipe to create a fat person: One part starvation plus one part stress. Throw in a heaping spoonful of inactivity. Blend until smooth. Take internally on a daily basis. In no time, you will be fat without trying!

Of course it's more complex than that. We promised no physiology lessons here. Biochemistry is a great sleep aid. Pick up a textbook if you are interested!

The last chapter covered the heaping spoonful of inactivity. The chapter before that discussed the role stress plays in how we feel. Now let's explore starvation. You might say, "I eat all the time! I'm far from starving!" Wrong. Let's check back in with *Oxford* for a moment. By definition, to starve is to "die or suffer acutely from lack of food; to feel very hungry." Hunger, according to the *Oxford Dictionary,* is "pain or discomfort felt when one has not eaten for some time; to have a strong desire for." Eating is the "act of chewing and swallowing food." (*Oxford* again!) OK. Food is a substance taken internally to maintain life. Eating is what we call that "taking in" process. Hunger is either a physical message that it is time to eat, or it is an emotional message of desire for something in particular. In order to successfully change your lifestyle forever, you must change your relationship with food. You must recognize when you are physically hungry and consume the substances your body needs to maintain life. You must recognize emotional hunger and satisfy that need with physical activity and any activity, other than eating that gives you pleasure.

What you eat is as important as when you eat. What kind of food does your body need to maintain life? It needs oxygen and water. Those are pretty basic foods. It also needs more complex foods, in the proper balance. You've heard it before, but it's worth repeating.

Your body needs the proper balance of protein, carbohydrates, fats, vitamins and minerals in order maintain life. The more natural the form of these building blocks, the more easily and completely they are utilized by the body.

Let's look briefly at *Oxford's* definition for "diet." We know it's a four-letter word, but let's look at it anyway just for a moment. Diet is defined as "the restricted selection of food." We ask this question: If food is essential for life, why restrict it? Not only does food restriction starve us of the essential nutrients our bodies need to live, but food restriction also makes us feel deprived. Nothing is pleasurable or likely to be repeated if it results in feelings of deprivation. Restricting food will just make the body want all the more of it. Food restriction leads to fatigue, which in turn encourages us to be more inactive. The more inactive we are, the weaker our muscles feel and the more fatigued we become. And the cycle continues. There are specific medical conditions that require restrictions of certain foods. Diabetes is a good example. Simple carbohydrates are restricted in order to maintain stable blood sugar levels. Everyone knows what happens to a diabetic who is out of balance. The diabetic can get circulatory problems resulting in loss of limbs, loss of essential organ function (kidney and heart especially), loss of sensation in the arms and legs and blindness. A person with atherosclerosis and/or coronary artery disease needs to restrict animal fats to reduce the amount of plaque buildup in the arteries and veins that lead to numerous problems, heart attack and stroke being some of the most serious.

Studies have shown that we begin to accumulate plaque in our arteries from the time we are two years old. With the current lifestyle so full of inactivity and fast food, is it no wonder that teenagers are having problems with high cholesterol? You have probably heard numerous references to the fact that our society is fatter than ever, despite all of the "fat-free" foods available. Another interesting fact is that the "average" woman is now considered to be 5' 4" tall and 140 pounds. "Average" is considered obese by many life insurance tables, and falls into the moderately obese category according to a well-known professional association. What is not always considered by may of these charts is the fact that this 5' 4", 140-pound female may not be overfat just because she is overweight. More and more women and men are taking care of themselves, getting regular activity and thereby building muscle. Let's take Melonie for example. She recently just zipped up her first pair of size 8 jeans. Melonie also weighs 134 pounds which falls into the moderately overweight category of many risk tables. Now give us your honest opinion. Would you really classify Melonie as moderately overweight? A size 8? According to all of those risk tables out there, we would need to weigh next to nothing, be anorexic, in order to fit in to their idea of a healthy weight!

Could this statement of the "average" be a ploy to get us to spend our hard-earned money on prescription drugs, special foods, and fat-free products? Do some of the various diet centers ever mention in their ads that their programs cause "starvation"? Do pharmaceutical companies openly tell you that their "miracle pill" that is supposed to help you lose weight may kill you in the process? (Some do now since their miracle drugs are starting to be banned in many states.) Do the manufacturers and distributors of all of those so-called fat-free "healthy foods" readily admit that the majority of their products contain just as much if not more sugar and sodium than their fat-containing counterparts? Not all of the diet centers, pharmaceutical companies and food manufacturers fail to consider safety and nutrition. The consumer needs to be educated. Knowledge is power!

With all of that being said, let's revisit the concept of starvation. Recalling the definition, starvation is to "die or suffer acutely from lack of food; to feel very hungry." Few of us are in danger of dying from the lack of food. Did you know your body could lapse into starvation mode if you exercise too much and don't eat enough? Yup, it can! Melonie explains her own experience with this concept:

> I had hit one of my many plateaus. No, let's rephrase that. Plateau is a diet word. Let's call it a "stall." I was stuck in this time warp for about three months, no more lost inches. I increased my calories to about 2,000 per day but continued to work very hard enjoying my activity breaks, racewalking six to seven miles per day, every day. Then Mother Nature took over. I strained both hamstrings, and had a terrible crushing injury to my big toe from a new pair of shoes (not my usual brand). Needless to say, I was sidelined from any activity for about a week. During that time, I could not walk. I did not reduce my caloric intake just because I was not as active. I continued to eat when hungry. After a week or so off, I was able to walk but not wear a shoe because of the toe. So, I bought a

larger size of cheap shoes and cut the toe out of one of them so I could start walking again. I was feeling so drugged out from lack of activity that it was driving me crazy. I had to slowly ease into my program, walking four to five miles every other day because of the hamstring injury. Guess what? I lost the four pounds I had gained several months prior. My legs healed. The toe took its own sweet time to heal. The moral of the story is, exercising too much can have the same effect as not eating enough.

The majority of us are in danger of becoming acutely ill from the lack of proper foods and over consumption of improper foods. A person could starve to death if she tried to live on table sugar alone. There is no nutritional value in table sugar. There is no protein. The carbohydrates are simple and metabolized quickly, leaving the circulating blood sugar even lower than it was just prior to consuming the table sugar. Table sugar contains no fat. Yes, we need some fat to live. Table sugar contains no vitamins or minerals. Now think of all of the foods we consume on a daily basis that contain table sugar. The next time you go to the grocery store, fill your cart as usual, then stop and read the labels. How many food products do not contain sugar? Don't be fooled by glucose, fructose, corn syrup, molasses, honey, etc. All of these and many other sweeteners are nothing more than various forms of table sugar. Most fruit juices contain added sugar. Double the whammy when it's concentrated. Sugar is still sugar. Sugar is added to pasta sauces, ketchup, soups, cereals, peanut butter, you name it. Sugar makes things taste good. Our society is one of sugar addicts!

We challenge you to live one day totally refined-sugar-free. You will find the majority of your food is in its natural state. You may have to make your own bread to have it be sugar free. You would consume meats, vegetables, fruits and legumes. Three out of four of those foods are high in fiber and low in fat. If you made your choices carefully, none of these foods would have been processed to death, having retained all of their natural fiber and nutrients. Are you beginning to see where we are going with this? You don't have to count calories or fat grams, or carbohydrate grams or protein grams. Whenever you eat a meal, have one-fourth be good quality protein (And that does not have to be meat!), one-fourth vegetables (raw or tender crisp preferred), one-fourth fruit (raw preferred, no juice), and one-fourth complex carbohydrates such as dried peas, beans and lentils, brown or wild rice, or any whole grain. We challenge you to find anything not of nutritional value in these foods. For those of you who have the need to deal with numbers, think about 30 percent protein, 10–20 percent fat, and the remainder of the percentage of calories coming from complex carbohydrate, with the majority of those being fruits, vegetables and whole grains. (These percentages are an example, a starting point, but may not be appropriate for everyone.)

Would you feel satisfied with this meal? One chicken breast, a large serving of seasoned brown and wild rice, green beans, two ears of corn swimming in butter, a large Caesar salad, and a pear or other fruit for dessert?

We are not proposing that you eat only unprocessed meat/protein, vegetables, fruits, legumes and whole grains, though we would all be healthier for it. What we are proposing is that foods in these quantities be the basis for your daily food consumption. If you are still hungry or have a craving, then supplement with whole grain bread and pastas rather than white flour products. Save floury baked goods and sweets for those times when you really crave them. Lay low with the tortilla chips and potato chips, even the baked varieties. Try to avoid using prepackaged entree mixes. The less foods have been processed, the more nutrients and fiber they retain, and the more satisfied you feel after eating them. Try this experiment. For breakfast one day, eat one serving of oatmeal made of whole or steel-cut oats, the kind you have to cook for twenty to thirty minutes. (Make it a day ahead, and rewarm it the next morning.) Top it with some fresh berries, cinnamon and applesauce or other fruit. Put some nonfat or skim milk on it if you like. Have a half cup of nonfat or low-fat cottage cheese, too. The next day, have the standard white or so-called wheat bread, topped with jam or jelly, and one so-called serving size of corn flakes or other standard cold cereal and perhaps some fruit. Which meal satisfied you more? Which stayed with you longer? The calorie counts were probably similar. There was likely more fat in the bread. Definitely more fiber in the oatmeal and fruit. For sure more refined sugar in the cold cereal and jam.

Here's the point. If you consume a diet that contains mostly processed, convenience foods, and do not consume enough fresh fruits and vegetables, your body will be starved of the essential nutrients it needs. You will feel fatigued, hungry, you may be more susceptible to illness, cuts may heal more slowly, hair and nails grow more slowly, skin becomes dry, you may suffer from allergies or skin problems. In summary, you just plain don't feel good and can't figure out why. Couple that with lack of activity and it's no wonder so many people are walking around so sick and tired of feeling sick and tired!

When Mel first started the food portion of her lifestyle change, she went whole hog, excuse the pun:

I had not consumed red meat for years, ever since all of the out-breaks of E.coli and hepatitis associated with improperly cooked meat at fast food restaurants. At that time, I ate a fast-food burger every work day for lunch, with fries of course! When that news hit the media, I immediately lost my taste for red meat and no longer trusted the foods prepared at fast food restaurants, and in many restaurants to be quite honest with you. When I first changed what fuel I gave my body, I went vegetarian. That is, I no longer ate meat, though I did consume dairy and eggs. I began to eat lots of pasta, beans and other legumes, bread, white rice, fruits and veg-etables. I also began to discover the fat-free foods filling the store shelves. I had read in one book that eating fat makes you fat, that by avoiding added fat in the diet, the body would be forced to use its own fat stores for the fat it needed to function.

Unfortunately, I did not heed the advice about limiting simple carbohydrates. I craved the fat-free chocolate goodies especially. I would consume an entire box of fat-free fudge brownies every three days. I had read I should eat bagels and pretzels when I got hungry. Of course, I was hungry every two hours. It seemed the more I ate like this, the more of these foods I wanted and the more hungry I felt. I was eating twice as many calories and was "starv-ing" all of the time. What my body was telling me was I was starving myself of quality food. I maintained this diet for the first year and a half. During this time, I did lose weight. I gained muscle mass. I also felt moody and had a hard time maintaining my en-ergy level. Then a stall came. My body would not increase its endurance or drop a pound. This went on for four months. I lapsed back into a more sedentary lifestyle, and started to feel like I had before the lifestyle change.

I then revisited my eating and activity patterns. I decided to cut out refined sugar entirely for one day, just as an experiment. Immediately, my energy level increased, my mood swings were gone. I had been experiencing daily headaches which did not occur the day I stopped the sugar. I felt less depressed, and much more relaxed. I felt so good, I decided to go for day number two. While I missed the chocolate brownies at first, I soon found myself craving them less. If I did get a craving, it was probably because of a lack of some chemical that occurs in chocolate, and I substitute fat-free, sugar-free instant chocolate fudge pudding or frozen yogurt. After the first month, I had not had one headache. I also had no PMS. I was sleeping the whole night through for the first time in years, and waking up feeling rested. I was finally convinced that refined sugar was poisoning me. Once I stopped the refined sugar, I had fewer cravings for other simple carbohydrates. Where pasta made with white flour used to be consumed at least daily, I now consume whole wheat pasta maybe once every two weeks. I find myself eating less white bread, and more brown rice and whole grains. I have not had or desired one of those fat-free fudge brownies in months. But watch out for the fat-free, sugar-free frozen yogurt in the summer! Of course, I indulge in my own versions of fudge brownies, lemon pie, cookies or a variety of other yummy things because I enjoy a bit of something sweet after a meal. I have just come up with ways to make my sweet treats treat my body sweetly, too!

When I reduced the amount of sugar I ate, the pounds began to come off almost effortlessly for several months. Just one other problem. I then began to crave peanut butter, and cheese, and cottage cheese, cream cheese, any kind of cheese, ice cream and meat. I thought, what's up? Then it dawned on me. I had eliminated most all of the fat in my diet. I was also not combining my non-meat proteins. My body was "starving" for protein and fat. As soon as I would eat a spoonful of peanut butter, a turkey sandwich, some fish or one-half small chicken breast, those cravings would stop and would not return for several days.

In contrast, let's take a look at how Jan began her foodstyle change:

I did not go whole hog. I finished off all of the high-fat stuff in my kitchen, gradually replacing it with lower-fat options. I did not experience intense food cravings. I did not change from a meat-and-potatoes girl to a vegetarian. I'm still a meat-and-potatoes girl. All I did was cut the fat. I, too, went through a time of being constantly hungry. But after I looked at my food intake, it was clear that my meals were balanced. Therefore, the reason I get hungry is because my body is getting well! It is coming out of starvation mode, realizing its hunger messages will be promptly addressed. My body needs more calories than what I was feeding it. The difference now is, it's waking up, getting very verbal and loudly demanding to be fed! Now that's true hunger. Once I started consuming enough of the right kinds of foods, that fat began to melt away.

So you see, no two people are alike. No two bodies react the same way to changes in food and activity levels. The one common thing we have discovered is that slow, gradual change causes less discomfort, physically and emotionally.

Balance. It's that simple. Feed your body what it wants, when it wants it, and in a reasonable quantity. Food cravings often signal the body's need for a certain type of fuel, whether it be protein, fat or a certain mineral.

Mel notices increased meat cravings when she is needing iron or protein.

I'm not sorry my eating habits evolved the way they did. Though I had not realized it, I had put myself on an elimination diet. By depriving my body of what it needed, I learned to recognize what the cravings meant. It took two years of ups and downs, plateaus and stressing out about my progress with fitness and weight loss, or lack thereof, before I finally discovered the simple solution. Balance.

Each person's body is unique. It has its own "comfortable" weight at which it wants to be. You cannot change what Mother Nature intended. Your goal should *not* be *just* losing weight. If you set a goal to feel better in three months, and use the tools of BodyLogic, you likely will feel better in three months, medical problems not withstanding, of course. If you set a goal to lose twenty pounds in three months, and starve yourself trying, you may or may not meet your goal, and you will feel sick and tired in the process. It is likely that your body will dine off of its lean muscle and continue to store even more fat because it thinks it's starving. The weight loss you get from starvation is mostly from loss of muscle and water. That's not healthy. That's not sane.

We mentioned before that your body does need some fat intake to survive. Fat contains fatty acids that help various processes in the body to work. You should be able to get enough fat in your diet just by eating the proper foods and in the right proportions. Notice we said *proportions* and not *portions!* You should not *have* to add any fat at all to your diet, unless you get as fat phobic as Mel did. If you don't eat meat, and most everything you buy is very low in fat or fat-free, and your body needs some 2,000 calories per day it may be difficult to even get 10 percent of calories from fat. Getting enough fat was difficult for Mel, and it still is. Too little fat (or too much fat!) has been shown to cause gallbladder disease, not to mention a variety of other ailments. The body does not produce most of the essential fatty acids found naturally in the foods we eat.

So what does a typical food day look like now? First of all, Mel still doesn't eat red meat. We don't eat high-fat foods, other than an occasional teaspoon or two of reduced-fat peanut butter on an English muffin when we really want it. Fried foods, pizza full of grease and rich desserts actually make us sick to our stomach. We get a headache and feel generally miserable until things, shall we say, "pass." We have also lost all liking and tolerance for alcohol. We just lost the taste for it; the desire for it even though Mel used to enjoy one glass of wine each evening after work.

I had not realized that I had the same bottle of wine in the fridge for over six months. I went to a party one night, and was served a Mai Tai. It looked kind of good, and everyone was in a festive mood. It took me two hours to get it down, and I was sick for the next two days. People have accused me of being compulsive about what I will or will not eat. They say I have such control. Such willpower. "How do you do it?" they ask. My reply? "I don't want to feel sick tomorrow." It's that simple. Most do not understand, and I do not expect them to. I just explain that I have intolerances to such foods. Somehow people understand a food allergy more than they do the concept of feeling well.

The alcohol? It lowers blood sugar and dehydrates you, and it slows metabolism—certain poison for a hypoglycemic or anyone who is trying to achieve steady blood sugar and promote fat-burning.

So then, a typical food day. We wake up in the morning and enjoy our coffee. Yes, caffeine is supposed to lower blood sugar and do all sorts of terrible things. But we do not react that way to it. We enjoy our two cups of coffee in the morning. They do not make us feel bad. Half an hour or so later, we eat a good, well-balanced breakfast. It usually consists of whole-grain pancakes with fruit and some cottage cheese, or English muffins or a bagel with fat-free cream cheese, fruit and yogurt, or maybe a vegetable and cheese omelet with some sort of bread and fruit. In the winter, we enjoy a hot bowl of oatmeal topped with unsweetened applesauce, sugar substitute and cinnamon. We try to avoid cereals that have a lot of sugar and are low in fiber. We are usually hungry again around 10:00 A.M. We have some fruit, and or whole-grain bread, or even a healthy toaster pastry or granola bar, or a fruit yogurt.

Lunch is between 11:30 and noon. We enjoy some vegetarian or turkey chili, a whole wheat pita with humus, or tuna salad made with water-packed tuna and fat-free mayo, maybe a grilled cheese sandwich or a tuna melt, a turkey sandwich, a vegetable pizza, a meatball sandwich, hot dogs or whatever we want (healthier versions, of course). We try to eat some hot veggies, or a salad, and some fruit. By 3:00 P.M. or so, hunger hits again. We have something similar to the morning snack. Mel's evening meal is usually an adventure.

I love Indian food, and will eat either vegetable or chicken curry. I also enjoy Thai stir-fried veggies, extra spicy. Sometimes it's chicken fixed one of a hundred different ways, or occasionally some whole-wheat pasta. I always have a salad, and/or veggies and fruit. I love spicy ethnic foods and have found ways to make low-fat versions of pizza, tacos, burritos, enchiladas, cheese "burgers" and many other things. Sometimes, I am totally lazy, and will just fix some steamed veggies or soup. It all depends on how hungry I am. When I eat a well-balanced lunch, I am less hungry in the evening. I drive people crazy when I pour hot sauce or cayenne pepper all over everything. One thing I discovered is when I reduced the fat, I found myself using spices to perk up the flavor. I must have burned out my heat receptors because I can usually tolerate more heat than anyone I am with. I have not gone so far as to begin eating jalapenos directly out of the jar, but I am sure that day is coming!

Jan tends to get into a rut with her evening meals.

My meals are not as adventurous as Melonie's. I usually eat a basic chicken breast, rice, vegetable and milk. I usually get home from work at 7:30 or 8:00 P.M., am hungry and don't want to take the bit of extra time necessary for creativity. I need to learn to plan ahead!

You may have noticed that we eat every two to three hours. Much of the literature shows that a person's metabolism is slowest early in the morning, especially a fat person's. Breakfast jump-starts that metabolism and activity keeps it going. We have also learned that it is better to spread your meals throughout the day, eating food every two to three hours, rather than consuming two or three larger meals. This keeps your blood sugar stable, and provides a constant source of fuel for your body. Another great benefit of eating frequent small meals is it keeps you from being so hungry that you overeat at meal time. Did you know it can take twenty to thirty minutes after some meals, especially low-fat ones, for your brain to register that you feel full? Here's a trick for you, especially if you tend to be a fast eater. Try eating your meals in courses, cooking one while eating the other. Here's an example:

Prepare a green salad and some sort of bread.

While eating the salad and bread, cook the vegetables.

By the time you are finished with the salad course, the veggies are ready.

While eating the veggies, put your entree on (either stove-top or in the microwave).

By the time the veggies are down, the entree is ready.

Then dive into the entree. If you find yourself full halfway through the entree, put what you don't eat in the fridge to reheat the next day for lunch or your evening meal.

Eating this way serves a couple of purposes. First, it forces you to eat slower, or at least over a longer period of time, giving your body time to register when it has had enough to eat. Second, it encourages you to consume your vegetables first, so if you fill up before you have finished your meal, you at least have your veggies for the day.

This style of eating works whether you are eating alone or dining with others. When dining with others, it allows more time for, guess what—communication! That's one major thing lacking in families these days. It seems the dinner table is used more for homework than it is for eating. Eating this way also instills healthy habits in other members of the family. It's a win-win for everyone. By the way, most of the recipes provided later in the book lend themselves to this way of eating.

Nighttime is often the worst for most of us. That's when the baseball game comes on or something else great on TV and you get the munchies. So what! Pretzels, low-fat popcorn, grapes or veggie sticks usually satisfy the need to munch. You might find that if you eat a high-fiber meal that includes protein around 6:00 or 6:30 P.M., you're not hungry in the evening. If you are munching because you are hungry, have some real food for a snack, such as a turkey sandwich, soup and an English muffin, some high-fiber cold cereal, fruit, yogurt, or whatever. If you are really not hungry, try to find something to busy your hands. That will get your mind off of the munchies. Keep a daily BodyLogic diary, work, do counted cross stitch, or practice a new skill such as oil painting. Keeping your mind on other things keeps it off food.

It is a good idea to have some complex carbo before bed, as your body will be going into a long fast until morning. That carbo snack helps keep the metabolism revved up a bit longer, and prevents you from waking up hungry in the middle of the night.

In later chapters, you will find sample menus for what we typically eat in a day, as well as samples of some of our favorite recipes that we have come up with. You will also find a substitution list, as well as "before and after" menus, to teach you how you can "have your cake and eat it too!" (Don't take that too literally.)

Don't cut your fat down too low. Fat does contain essential fatty acids needed by the body to function. The majority of these fatty acids are not produced by the body. Stick to mono- and polyunsaturated sources of fat. Fat helps you feel fuller longer, and it keeps things moving along through the digestive tract, as does fiber. But even with all the fiber we eat, we notice if our fat intake is too low, we will have problems occasionally.

Everyone is different, and some of us are habitually addicted to regiment. We must count every carbohydrate, fat and protein gram, and of course every calorie. That's OK. The difference is now you do it to make sure you are getting a balanced diet and eating enough, not to measure how deprived you feel today. One other thing we must tell you if you really want to take care of yourself is to repeat what we said earlier, and that is you must change your relationship with food. *Never say the words good, bad, and food in the same sentence* unless you are describing a flopped recipe! Your self-worth is not and cannot be measured by the kind of food you eat. You are not a good or bad person because you ate fruit versus peanut butter. You are a good person, and food is a necessary thing that you can enjoy. Stop the negative self talk. Don't expect to make major changes overnight. Start small and work up. If you want to feel good for life, you must proceed in logical, progressive steps. That's BodyLogic!

We said it before, and we will say it again and again until you get it: Food is fuel. Eating too much fat will make you fat. But if you are really hungry, and you are eating all of the right things, don't stress about counting calories! Stop being afraid of food. Just eat. Eat enough to keep your body out of starvation mode.

All this talk about food and calories we're sure has you asking, "OK, sounds fine, but how much am I supposed to eat?" Everyone is different. You have to eat enough to provide your body with the minimum amount of fuel and nutrients it needs just to maintain its functions, not to mention whatever activities you do or stress you are under. The goal with all of this is *not* losing weight! It *is* about gaining health! Weight is relative. It is a number on a scale that really does nothing other than generate revenue for scale manufacturing companies, the diet industry and life insurance companies not to mention making you feel bad when that number goes up. Every part of your body weighs something. Bones are heavy. Muscles weigh something. Skin and organs weigh something. Then you add all the fluid on board. What's left is fat, and you need some of that too to protect your organs, keep you warm and allow for certain body functions on a chemical level. Too much will kill you.

Achieving a healthy body is about *losing fat and gaining muscle*. Losing fat is not as important as gaining muscle in how you feel. With increased muscle mass, you move better, you have more energy and you feel better. Ever wonder why a 400-pound person can barely walk across the room? Not enough muscle to carry the fat weight! We have seen fit people who are overfat. That's OK, too. For those of us who have been overfat all of our lives, the body may refuse to let go of its fat. So be it. But it will feel better, move better and live longer if its muscles, including the heart muscle, are strong, and it is given enough quality fuel to function in a healthy way. The people who are morbidly overfat and cannot lose fat by any means are really few and far between. So don't immediately say, "I'm one of those, I will never lose fat." NEVER SAY NEVER! If you build muscle and eat quality food and consume a diet low in fat, your muscles will use the fat stored to function between meals and during times of increased activity or stress. It's not so much the calories, but the kind of calories.

Forget about what everyone has told you. You know the formula: If calories in are less than calories out, you will lose weight. If calories in are greater than calories out, you will gain weight. We are living proof this is not true. Mel remembers when she was at her maximum weight.

I continued to breathe on 800–1,300 calories per day but I certainly was not living. At that weight, leading a sedentary lifestyle, my body needed 1,500–1,900 calories to get the nutrients it needed just to make ends meet. I literally force-fed myself to reach that intake, and low and behold, I started losing fat. A good friend of mine is the same height, weighs four pounds more, but wears one to two sizes smaller than I do. How can that be? Her "weight" is muscle, lean muscle. She has a very low body fat percentage. She runs at least three times per week, covering seven miles per hour. Her bones are smaller than mine as well. So I know that based on my frame size, it probably isn't realistic to expect that I will ever wear the same size that she does. So what! I have gone from a size 24 Woman's to a size 8 Petite. My legs are hard as rocks. If I increase my exercise and my calories, I will gain a couple of pounds. So what! I'm still losing inches. That means those extra couple of pounds are muscle weight, and that's a good thing, because when I'm doing nothing, those muscles will burn my body fat for fuel when nothing else is around.

We're telling you here and now, this is the only day that you will ever step on that scale again. After today, throw it out, and don't buy another one. *The scale lies.* We'll say it again: *The scale lies!* Post that message everywhere and never forget it. If a shrinking body is something you want to watch happen, measure yourself (after your period if you are still menstruating) and watch yourself buy progressively smaller sizes in clothing. Better yet, get your body fat percentage tested, then don't do it again for a year or so. Then retest. We can almost guarantee you if you follow this plan your fat percentage will drop. If you maintain or gain "weight" with a lower body fat percentage, that means you are adding lean muscle, not fat. Better yet, measure success and wellness by how you feel, how you sleep, how much energy you have, how shiny your hair is and that healthy glow to your skin. We are firm believers that you can be even moderately overfat (but not morbidly) and improve your health at the same time. Your body has an astute awareness as to what it needs to feel good. Listen to it and give it what it needs. If you do that, fat loss will come as a secondary benefit. Just don't expect to look like an anorexic cover model. Who wants to?

All weight is not created equal! Don't ever forget it. We will stop preaching now. We learned these concepts the hard way, through a lot of emotional pain. If we can keep you from going through all of that, then his book has served its purpose.

Finally, as we move forward, you will find what we hope to be some very humorous moments. We want you to laugh. We both have a sense of humor and appreciate each other's. We will talk to you as we talk to each other. You must learn to laugh at some of those things in life that bring you discomfort. It is a way of coping. It also helps you to readjust your thinking, make positives out of negatives, and realize that there are people out there whose problems are much worse than yours. Be happy with yourself. Laugh at yourself. Take care of yourself, because you are the only you that will ever be! Don't ever try to be like someone you are not.

> ***Your positive self statement for today: I am strong, and powerful, and in control of my body!***

Fuel-Style Overhaul Time!

Increasing Miles per Gallon, or Energy Efficient Fuel

Here we go. Now we start the "how to." This is *our* how-to. It is not just about losing weight or losing fat! It's about being healthy. And it is presented to give you the tools to develop *your* how-to. For example, Mel hates beef, you may love it; but, you will find adaptations to reduce the fat in your typical style of preparing that beef. You know what they say about people in third-world countries. Give them the tools to grow their own food and they will survive. Make them dependent on others and they won't survive. In the next several chapters we will be providing information on menu structuring, tips, recipes, sample menus, and menu make-overs, as well as fat, protein, carbohydrate and calorie counts for many of *our* favorite foods. Take these tools, adapt them, and come up with your own foodstyle.

Our intent is not to make your life regimented. If you become regimented about eating, you are in that old diet mentality and your thoughts will habitually return to "what more can I eat today" rather than "what more do I need to eat today"? Decisions about whether or not to give your body fuel will be based on hunger. Hunger is your body's fuel gauge. That's BodyLogic. Unfortunately (or fortunately) depending on how you look at it, some structure is necessary for BodyLogic freshmen, like yourselves. Once you have achieved your first goal or each time you encounter a stall, you may need to re-evaluate your body's needs. Perhaps illness or injury makes you more inactive, you are not feeling as good as you used to, the addition or a loss of someone in the household or some other life stressor causes a relapse in the old way of thinking.

You must walk before you can run. You must tolerate running one mile before you can run three, and in order to run three you might have to modify how you ran that one-mile stretch. Life is ever changing. Your body's needs are ever changing. Once these concepts become habit, you will no longer need the structure until something in your life changes that triggers the need to reevaluate or modify the changes you made previously. It's like painting your bathroom. Once you learn to slap on the paint in the traditional manner, you won't need the how-to guides anymore. But if you decide you are bored with that bathroom, and want to try a different technique like sponge painting, you need to pull that manual out and learn the additional steps involved. The basics probably haven't changed much, but a few new steps have been added or maybe the kind of paint you use will need to be changed. Instead of using only a paintbrush, now you use a paintbrush and a sponge. BodyLogic works the same way. You never stop learning, you never stop achieving new things, you never stop growing and you never stop changing.

First things first. You must start with the basics. While parts of this chapter may seem laborious and highly structured, they are part of your learning process. Many of these exercises will only have to be done a few times. Once mastered, you will have the tools to start changing not so much what you eat, but the way you eat.

First you must learn how much fuel your body needs, like estimating how much paint you will need for that bathroom make-over. You need to calculate the approximate daily caloric need for your weight based on activity level. Think of it like planning your next car trip. Let's say you face a three-hour drive. The first thing you do is check the gas gauge. You know how far your car can go on a tank of gas, and you fill the tank accordingly. If the tank is already nearly full, likely you will not top it off. You must learn to fuel your body in the same way.

The intent of the caloric or fuel-need formula is to give you a range of fuel intake to keep you healthy. These numbers are not carved in stone and certainly will not fit everyone's needs. Things like age, height, muscle mass and sex must also be factored in. Now is not a time for denial or deception. If you see stuff on your body that is hanging, rolling and flopping around, the majority of your weight is not muscle. If you flex your leg and cannot see the "cut" of muscle, the majority of your weight is not muscle. If you don't know what "cut" is, turn on the TV and watch men (or women) engaging in some sort of athletic activity. As they move their bodies, their muscles contract, and you see the shape or cut of those muscles as they move. The easiest, but most unrealistic example of cut is to watch a body-building competition. You will see more cut than you ever thought possible, and may discover a few extra hormones you didn't know you had! Don't stress out. One day soon, you will start to feel the muscle. Later, you will start to see the muscle.

Start by weighing yourself. Yes, the scale must be used on occasion. Best to use a friend's or one away from home and throw out your own scale. And don't be like Mel and run out and buy another one—actually she bought two. One frustration for the woman over 300 pounds is that the height/weight charts (and most doctor's scales!) only go to 300 pounds. Who set that magic number? It may be a challenge to find a scale that will weigh you, but the effort will be worth it. You may need to go to a rental place that has heavy duty scales, rent one for a day, and take care of business! If you have a medical school near you, or a teaching or research hospital, give a call and see if they have a scale you could use from time to time for an accurate weight check. Ask your doctor to order extra weights for the clinic's scale so you and others can have a "known" with which to work. Or, at home, use two bathroom scales. Place one foot on each and total the numbers. If you cannot find a scale, do not become obsessed with it. Use the fact that you weigh more than 300 pounds as a benchmark. You will need to make an honest best-guess as to your weight. For example, you probably know how many pounds up or down necessitates a change in the size of your clothes. Think back to the last time you could weigh on a standard scale and think about what size you were then versus what size you are now. You are probably a better judge of your weight than you think.

There are hundreds of different versions of height/weight charts that give varying numbers of recommended caloric intake based on body-frame size. Look hard enough and you will find one with which you might agree. This has been one of our greatest frustrations, to determine how many calories we need to get adequate nutrition based on varying degrees of activity? Out of frustration, Mel came up with a simple formula that should put most of you within the ballpark, probably about a 400-calorie spread from the minimum to the maximum. If you "don't do math," that's OK, too. We have included a chart at the end of the book with many of the numbers calculated for you. If you are 5' 5" or less, look to the lower end of the range. If you are 5' 6" or more, lean toward the higher end. If you have been overfat for the majority of your life, look toward the lower end. If you have been overfat for only a few years, look to the higher end. These numbers are not precise, but they will put you within a good range in which to start. Adjust up or down by 100 calories or so depending on how you feel and how your clothes are fitting over the first twelve weeks. If you notice an uptrend in clothing size or an increase in your measurements from the eight-week mark on, cut back calories some, or better yet increase activity by fifteen to thirty minutes a day if you can tolerate it. Experiment with increasing activity then increasing or decreasing calories. The goal is to have enough energy to get through the day and then some, and not be hungry more often than every three hours or so. Don't forget it takes a minimum of six weeks to get out of starvation mode for most people. It took Mel eight to ten weeks. A lot depends on how long you have been torturing your body. Your body's initial response to BodyLogic may be to continue to store fat, until it is convinced that the days of starvation are long over. Once your mind convinces your body of that, the changes you want will start to happen. Healing takes time. Be patient! You have all the time in the world!

Remember that a balance in your food intake is key. Living on carbs without enough protein or fat will leave you hungry all of the time, and you will end up eating more than your body probably needs. However, if you are eating the right balance of foods, and are hungry all the time, give yourself permission to eat! Everything will balance out in time.

Use this time to learn what is right for *your* body, not what some expert says. (Nothing against experts, but every "body" is different!) That is the whole concept behind BodyLogic. Don't ever feel forced to fit into someone else's box or idea of what a healthy eating and activity plan is. Develop your own, based on what your individual needs, likes and dislikes are.

First, look at the following list and estimate honestly your average daily activity level:

1) I sit or lie down all day, and do nothing but eat and care for bodily functions. (The level similar to your activity if you are in a hospital.) (0)

2) I sit most of the day, I don't exercise, and I don't do strenuous household or recreational activities. I may have an office job and do light housework. Most of my walking is from the car to the store or office, and sum total probably is not more than 30–60 minutes per day at a casual stroll. I spend time each day sewing, doing light gardening or similar activities. (Consider an activity level like playing pool. Lots of stop and go, stop and go, never really going very fast and not getting very far—unless you are winning of course!) (200)

3) I may have a desk job but I am always away from my desk, or I am a professional shopper or a chef. I'm on my feet most of the day between work and household chores. I walk or ride a bike or engage in some light physical activity 3–4 times per week. I can walk 3.5 miles in an hour comfortably and do it regularly, or I ride my bike covering about 5 mph. (500)

4) I have a fairly active job. I may be a housekeeper or do professional lawn care. I may do a lot of lifting and walking at my job. I may be a nurse who is lifting patients and on my feet all day long and/or I participate in strenuous physical activity 6–7 days per week, and lift weights, racewalk, jog, run, use a rowing machine or a ski machine, or swim laps, or a combination of similar activities. (We consider this level for BodyLogic alumni!) (900)

Let's use Mel being sedentary as the base for your calculation. You will use this same formula each time you reevaluate how much energy your body needs. Get out some paper, a pen and a calculator. Here we go!

At 140 pounds (Actually 134, but we made it easy!), height 5' 4" and her activity level is 1.

Start by writing down 1,500 calories. That is Mel's basic need for activity level 1, and your starting point from here on out.

For each 10 pound increase in weight over 140 pounds, add 130 calories, PLUS

For activity level 1, no calculation.

For activity level 2, add 200 calories.

For activity level 3, add 500 calories.

For activity level 4, add 900 calories.

This will give you your ballpark caloric need.

Here's an example. Let's say Mel is in the level 4 activity category (which she is most of the time! Yes, she still needs BodyLogic to keep her on track!)

Here's the math: Base = 1,500 calories. Don't add for weight. Add 900 calories for activity level 4. This puts her needs at 2,400 calories, or a range of 2,200–2,600. When Mel eats right and listens to her body, she consumes 2,000–2,200 calories per day without gaining fat and while slowly losing inches. As Mel is 5' 4" tall she leans toward the lower end of the range. In addition, because she has been fat all of her life, her metabolism will probably never reach a "normal" level. Perfecto! Some days are hungry, she eats more. Some days are not hungry, she eats less. The secret is feeling satisfied, eating when hungry, not gaining fat, and losing inches. This means you are re-placing fat with muscle. Muscle is heavy. *The scale lies*! Measure in terms of what you gain!

OK. Let's do one a bit harder.

Let's say Mel went off the deep end, or broke her leg or some-thing. She now weighs 150 and is only at an activity level 2. *("Hey, I never could use crutches! If I could, I'd probably be at a level 3 on the activity scale!")* Here's the math.

Base = 1,500 calories.

Add 130 calories for each 10 pounds in weight over 140. 1,500 + 10 pounds divided by 10 x 130= 1630. Add 200 calories for activity level 2. 1500 + 130+ 200 = 1830. Mel's range is probably 1,630–2,030 calories per day, depending on how active she is at her level 2.

Now for a harder one. Still use Mel, only this time the "Mel before BodyLogic."

Weight 220. Activity level 1. She hated to move and she didn't have to very much!

Base = 1,500. Now add 130 calories for each 10 pounds over 140. That calculation is 80 pounds divided by 10 x 130 = 1040. The total is: 1,500 + 1,040 = 2,540. At that time, Mel needed to eat between 2,300 and 2,700 calories to get what her body needed to function. "When I hit rock bottom, I had really cut back on the food, and guesstimated I was consuming maybe 1,000 to 1,300 calories a day if I was lucky. Was I starving? Yup! Couldn't tell it by looking at me back then!"

Let's do one that might more closely resemble the woman this book is written for. Let's say we have a person weighing 240 pounds, with a desk job at an activity level 2.

Base = 1,500. Now we add 130 calories for each 10 pound increase in weight over 140 pounds. That's 100 pounds divided by 10 = 10 x 130 = 1,300. Now add 200 calories for activity level 2. Add all that up: 1,500 + 1,300 + 200 = 3,000 calories. This woman would need between 2,800 and 3,200 calories just to keep her body healthy!

OK. Here's another one.

A 325-pound woman who runs her own business but doesn't regularly exercise. Her job is part at the desk, and part on her feet. (I bet you know by now who this person is, or at least used to be!) Probably on the high end of a level 2 on the activity scale.

Base = 1,500. We add 130 calories for each 10 pounds over 140. That's 185 divided by 10 x 130 = 2,405. Now we add 200 calories for that activity level 2. 1,500 + 2,405 + 200 = 4,105. This woman could conceivably need 3,900–4,300 calories to keep her body out of starvation mode and maintain her health as well as her weight. Now, if that woman went to a doctor or a diet center to ask for help with losing weight, what would happen? She likely would be put on a calorie count half as much lower than what she needs to be healthy (unless she is lucky and has a very smart doctor!)

OK. Let's do one more. Let's say this lady weighs 425 pounds. She does not work outside of the home. She spends her day in front of the TV, dreaming about being a few pounds less so she can have energy for at least a part-time job. Let's face it, there is weight discrimination out there! We put her at an activity level 1.

Here's the math: Base = 1,500. Add 130 calories for each 10 pounds over 140. That's 285 divided by 10 x 130 or 3,705. There is no calculation for activity level 1. The calculation is: 1,500 + 3,705 = 5,205! Her range is likely between 5,000 and 5,400 calories! Let's face it, she most likely is not healthy at her present weight, and to be realistic, needs to be under a doctor's care while attempting to change her lifestyle. She will need special activities like water aerobics or something she can pedal while sitting in a chair in order to increase her fitness level enough to start losing some fat so her muscle can move her around more easily. She needs to eat the right kind of food and the right amount of it. Again, she must be under a doctor's care. The case of this woman is probably much less frequent than the ladies we looked at before, but it is included to show you the trend of weight versus nutritional need.

OK. Now it's *your* turn. Mark this page and use a pencil so you can refer back to it whenever you want or need to (we have also included some extra worksheets in the back of the book):

Base = :   1,500 calories

Add 130 calories for each 10 pounds over 140 pounds:

+_____

(Your weight minus 140 divided by 10 x 130)

Add your activity factor (see the numbers in the list above):

+_____

And the grand total is: _____

Your range is approximately 200 less to 200 calories more than the grand total:_____   See the trend? The more you weigh and the more active you are, the more fuel your body needs to stay healthy. Not all fuel is created equal. We will explain more about that later.

For now, if your caloric intake falls much below the range you calculated, recheck your math and make sure you were honest about your weight and activity level. After all, this is about being true to yourself. You only cheat yourself by not being honest. If all of that checks out, your body is likely in starvation mode. Instead of burning fuel for energy, it is storing quite a bit of it as fat, trying to store enough fuel to keep you breathing, but not much else! If it is taking in lots of fat through meals, there is no reason to use what is stored. To slow down this fat storage process and increase the utilization of the food you eat for fuel, you must eat enough calories and in the right proportions. You must increase your metabolism to burn more fuel. Your body will figure out the rest once it believes it is not going to starve to death. Remember, too little fuel and/or too much activity will have the same effect—starvation mode and fat storage. Too little activity and too much fuel will either increase body fat percentage or it will result in maintenance at a high fat percentage, like Jan explained in her story.

Next, you need to do an exercise in self-exploration and face some cold hard facts. Before you start developing your own customized program, you need to establish baselines. Start with your measurements. One hundred twenty-inch measuring tapes are available through BodyLogic. (Use the order from in the back of the book.) Have a photo taken (a full-body shot), videotape yourself, draw your current silhouette on a full length mirror and identify some reference point for activity (e.g. "I can walk one-half block comfortably.") Find one pair of pants that fit perfectly, mark them in some way and never get rid of them. Keep a food diary for at least two weeks. Write down the exact quantities of foods that you eat and when you eat them. Make note of what you are feeling at the time. Is it really hunger? Stress? Boredom? Keeping up with the Jones' at a party? Whenever possible, indicate calories, carbos, protein and fat grams. Don't judge yourself during this time. This will be the beginning of a very important tool for you. Don't try to "be good." Don't change your current food intake at all. Live as you have been, eat as you have been, but write down every bite and the totals.

At the end of the first two weeks of your diary, calculate the total daily average of calories. Add up the calories for each day and divide by fourteen days. Now, compare this with the number you calculated. If your intake is greater than the number you calculated, you need to decrease calories to give your body what it needs without giving it any extra. If your intake is lower than the one you calculated, make sure you estimated correctly. If so, start eating more quality food. Note: The emphasis here is on "quality. "Go somewhere around half way between your present intake and the maintenance intake. Most likely your body is in starvation mode, and it needs to be gradually made aware that the famine is over! Don't worry if you think you have gained a few pounds during this time (Did you throw out the scale yet?) Now you have a starting point.

Before you get excited (or depressed as the case may be) keep in mind that all calories are not the same. Some get used more efficiently by the body than others do: 1 gram of protein equals 4 calories. One gram of carbohydrate equals 4 calories. One gram of fat equals 9 calories. Fat is stored first and used for energy last. Fat is what you see on your body, what makes you jiggle and what causes those rolls under your clothes. It's what makes your thighs rub together and gives you rashes or other irritations where skin rubs on skin. It's what makes your breasts sag and belly drag! Fat has only a trace of essential nutritional value in comparison to protein and carbohydrate.

Fat does provide some essential fatty acids your body needs that it cannot produce on its own, but you will likely get enough fat from eating the right foods without having to add any extra. (If you are like Mel and totally fat phobic, then you need to watch to make sure you get enough of the right kind of fat.) So, the bottom line is this. If you cut back on fat, you get to eat more food to get the same number of calories. We wouldn't call that deprivation or starvation! What would satisfy you more, two tablespoons of peanut butter or a large low-fat whole wheat bagel with fat-free cream cheese? If you had missed lunch and were really hungry, and could have one or the other to last you for the next four hours, which would you choose? Would you be more satisfied with two tablespoons of oil or two cups of fat-free refried beans or a bagel with fat-free cream cheese? Trust us. Eat the beans or the bagel, and watch the fat on your body disappear. Imagine the rush of blood carrying vital nutrients to all of your organs through unclogged pipes. The body will use what it has to meet its need for fat, at least for the majority of the people.

Here's a little more experience talking from Melonie:

While writing this book, I hit a major stall and could not figure out why I was gaining fat while exercising more, and why I was "starving" all of the time. If I had listened to my body, when I said to myself, "Why am I starving all of the time," I would have had my answer. I was literally starving! As it turns out, I took a hard look at my foodstyle again. I was trying to live on 1,300 calories/day, power walking 60–90 minutes per day (a good 600–800 calorie burn), which meant there were only 500 calories left over to maintain my bodily functions and build muscle at the same time. You can only overdraw the checking account just so much before you become aware of it. More analysis found I should be consuming anywhere from 2,100–2,500 calories per day. My fat intake was also only 2 percent of calories from fat. That is not healthy. No one should go below 10 percent of calories from fat. Ten to 30 percent is the recommended range. (The more body fat you have to lose, the higher your risk for heart disease and stroke, the lower the fat percentage should be.) So I started eating 1,800–2000 calories per day, started making sure I got enough fat and guess what? I gained a couple of pounds. I know, I said throw out the scale. This is the one time where I will say, "Don't do as I do, do as I tell you!" Then a few injuries hit which sidelined me for a couple of weeks. During that time, I could only walk every other day, and only five miles instead of six to seven. Know what happened while I was eating more and exercising less? My leg measurements started to increase. Don't think: *Oh she is backsliding.* Not so. My body was readjusting to eating again, continuing to store some fat while it came out of starvation mode. You know what happened during next several weeks? Arm measurements became smaller, as did waist, hips, thighs and unfortunately, chest. So fat was finally burning. Within a couple of more weeks of listening to my hunger signals, I was averaging 2,000–2,100 calories per day and I had lost about a pound of what I had gained. So the starvation mode was reversing! There was no muscle pain and my muscle bulk continued to increase. So I know I am burning fat! What did I learn from this stall? My body was working hard to maintain itself while I was inadvertently torturing it. I also learned that I do not have to move my body at a high intensity every day, and in fact I should not. That's what causes injuries. I learned my lesson.

The body does not use up its fat in a fair and equitable manner. It may decide to dine on the right thigh instead of the left for a while, then it will move to the belly and forget about the thigh. It may linger over the double chin or even dine on the feet. For some inhumane reason, it saves the best for last, usually the belly and thighs. Must be gold in there! The smallest areas of the body will shed their fat first. The larger areas will be the last to change. It all averages out over time, so don't get discouraged. Of more importance is how you feel. In starvation mode, you have no energy to move. You find yourself being able to walk less and less, and at a slower and slower pace. Your muscles hurt, you may have trouble sleeping. Your mind slows down and you cannot concentrate. As soon as you start eating again, you will feel more inclined to move your body. Once you do, your fitness level will rapidly increase. You might start sleeping less but feeling much more alert. We kid you not. The brain functions on glucose (sugar), and functions best when its glucose comes from complex carbohydrates rather than refined sugar. Would that *Concord* keep going if all of its fuel tanks were empty? We don't think so.

How long would your car run on fumes before it finally quit? Get out of the diet mentality and start living. Do it in a logical way.

Time to fatten up your garbage can (or your friends!)

The next step of the program is to defat your kitchen. Keep in mind that your lifestyle change will be as healthy for your family as it is for you, and with a few simple tricks, the family will never miss the fat. And if you are fortunate enough to start when the kids are young, you will be instilling in them good nutritional habits that will last a lifetime, and prevent them from having to go through the humiliation of obesity or the pain and disability of heart disease, diabetes, stroke or a myriad other disorders.

Mel explains her experience with life after she found BodyLogic like this:

> One thing I have had the pleasure of learning while going through my lifestyle change is this: Being a good role model changes the way other people live too! Time after time of dining out with friends, they see what food choices I make. Over the past few years, I have noticed them making healthier choices, even if they have no particular goals other than to maintain their present level of health, whatever that may be. The majority of my friends are now fat phobic, but many continue with their sugar addictions.

> The other night I went out to dinner with some friends, one of whom I had not seen for several years. She was totally shocked when I walked in the door of the restaurant. I was about a size 18 the last time we got together. From the time I sat down, she watched my every move, from what I ordered (linguini with red sauce with all kinds of seafood, spinach salad and sourdough bread), to what I left on the plate. (Bacon from the salad. I hate bacon!) By the end of the meal, she said, "You have given me the inspiration I need to get my life on track. From here on out, I'm going to make time for me and care for myself as I should." One small step for humans; one giant step for humankind!

> You know, it's really funny. Lately I've noticed when I eat with a group of people, after I order my meal, others who order after me will select healthier choices and those who have already placed their order will ask for the dressing on the side, or dry toast, or whatever after the fact. It's as if they feel guilty eating what I chose not to have! Oh, if they could only think about it differently.

So your healthy choices will eventually have an impact on the worst double-cheeseburger addict you have ever met, even if they only downscale to a regular cheeseburger, it's still a step in the right direction. If you have family in the house, be sneaky how you prepare food. Start with having the fried chicken skinned before you fry it, then move on to oven fried. Change from whole milk to 2 percent, then 1 percent, then skim. Switch from Half & Half to a mixture of one part Half & Half to one part milk, then to whole milk then phase down. Do the same thing with all of your dairy products and higher-fat foods. It's kind of like the cost of a postage stamp. You notice a 15 cent raise more if it comes all at once, rather than in 2 or 3 cent increments. The end result is the same, but it's much less painful getting there. The same concept is applied to any part of a lifestyle change.

Start with small changes, then increase gradually to have an end result that is very different from the beginning, but without feeling deprived.

If you live alone, or have only one other person in the house who wants to make the same changes as you, and if you are a strong person, you can defat the kitchen all at once. For Mel, it was kind of a cathartic, a way of saying "good-bye" to the old lifestyle and "hello" to the new one. She spent an entire Saturday in the kitchen, (not to mention the bedroom, the office, the car, even the bathroom! Yes, food was everywhere!) with several large trash bags and boxes. She went through every cupboard, the pantry, the fridge and the freezer and got rid of everything that had more than 3 grams of fat per serving, with the exception of her peanut butter.

You must defat your kitchen. You can do it all at once like Mel, or you can do it gradually like Jan. It does not matter just as long as you do it and pronto. If you choose the gradual route, give yourself a target date. Each time you run out of a high-fat food, make the next purchase a version of the same food only lower in fat. If that's not possible, select an appropriate substitution. Make a list of those things you don't think you could do without: cooking oil, cheese, cold cereals, frozen dinners, canned tuna, salad dressing, pasta sauce, etc. Make a second list of foods that bring you pleasure but need to have some healthier substitutions for: cookies, candy, muffins, potato chips, microwave popcorn, chocolate flavor creamer for your coffee, etc.

Keep one food for which there is no substitute, one food that brings you more true pleasure (not comfort) than any other. For Mel it was her chunky peanut butter! You might fully expect to have to replace your entire food supply.

What's left when you are finished may be astonishing: rice, pasta, beans, dried peas, several cold cereals, most breads, fruits and vegetables, turkey, chicken and the list goes on and on. Box up those things you know some friends (or enemies if you don't want to kill off your friends with all that fat!) would use and make the rounds the same day delivering all of your gifts of poor health. So should you tell your friends why you are giving away all of this food or should you keep it to yourself? That's up to you. Melonie handled her foodstyle change this way: "I told them I was making a few changes, cleaning out and could no longer use these things. I didn't say why. For me, broadcasting to the world my intent to change would mean total embarrassment if I failed. At that point in time, I did not realize that I already had succeeded and failure was pretty much impossible if I kept true to myself. I only told a few trusted friends, those whom I knew would be my support and not try to talk me into unhealthy choices."

People mean well, but often they don't understand what harm their words can do. "You can have one piece of cheesecake, it won't hurt you." "I slaved all day to prepare this meal, the least you can do is try it." "You will upset her if you don't eat." You might want to be selective about with whom you share your goals. You might also want to avoid any food situation that you might have difficulty dealing with until you have changed your lifestyle and grown personally enough to be able to say "No thank you. I can't tolerate that much fat. It makes me sick." "No thank you, I have a sensitivity to refined sugar." "No thank you, I don't drink." "No thank you, I already ate." And the statement that really shows you have made it: "No thank you, I'm not hungry!"

Simple statements like these are much better received than saying "I can't, I'm on a diet." Which statement would make you feel more deprived and alone in your pursuit of health? By now, you have freed yourself of the old diet mentality. Be aware that other people around you may not have achieved this level of personal growth. Be prepared for others to have you under their magnifying glass, fully prepared to make statements of dissatisfaction at the drop of a hat. Have more concern for yourself and your body than you do about the feelings of others. Just be polite. The feelings of satisfaction will be much greater than what a piece of chocolate cheese cake could ever provide. In time, you won't even think twice about going out to dinner at a friend's home and worry what you will eat when all that is served is meat lasagna with cheese, garlic bread loaded with butter, and a high-fat Caesar salad. You will have avoided the situation by politely asking what is on the menu. One trick is to say, "I hope you are not going to a lot of trouble fixing this meal. What can I bring to go with it?" Likely, your hostess will say, "Oh, it's just meat lasagna, I made it a day ahead." Politely insist on bringing a side dish or two, or perhaps the salad made with your own fat-free Caesar dressing, even the garlic bread made your way. That way, you can enjoy your visit, eat some of that lasagna, lots of the salad and a slice or two of bread, and only be half sick to your stomach! The next couple of days you watch your fat intake and go on with life as usual. The hostess is not upset, you are not deprived, and you have not totaled your body completely. Next time, you play hostess and invite those friends over for a gourmet feast that is healthier. We promise that with some practice, they won't know the difference. They will be amazed when they ask for the recipe!

The labels lie, sort of

Here's the skinny on fat. Fat is in almost everything. Fat is an inefficient fuel source. Fat is needed by the body in very small amounts. Too much fat collects in places you can see, but more importantly, it collects in places you can't see. All of the blood vessels. This restricts the flow of blood thereby depriving all of your organs of the oxygen and nutrients they need to function properly. When the heart does not get enough blood, a part dies. This is a heart attack. When the brain does not get enough blood, a part dies. This is a stroke. When the liver, kidneys and pancreas do not get enough blood, portions of them die. The eventual end result is liver failure, kidney failure and diabetes. Other things cause these disorders, but clogged arteries are the worst culprit. Are you starting to see the connection between life and fuel? Between fat intake and health? *So what if you don't lose a pound! Your body will still be healthier. Is that such a great disappointment?*

So how do you find the amount of fat in the food you eat?

Pull out your calculator, some paper and something with which to write. Yup. More math. You can skip the calculator if you have a high IQ for numbers. Here is the number-one thing you need to learn. Post this all over your kitchen, put it in your wallet, wherever it will be handy when you want to check the food you plan to buy or eat. Once you do this several times with various brands, you will develop a standard shopping list as well as sample restaurant choices so you won't have to keep doing this labor-intensive exercise forever, and no one will see you obsessing about your food.

Percentage of calories from fat=the number of fat grams in one serving, multiplied by 9, then divided by the number of calories in one serving.

Nutrition facts

Here are three examples of common foods and the calculations showing the amount of fat actually contained in them. Facsimiles of the nutrition labels from the packaging are shown so you can see how the information is presented to you and how you can work the math to see just what you are actually getting.

Let's start with "reduced-fat peanut butter." The label indicates that it contains 12 fat grams times 9 calories per gram equals 108 calories from the fat in one serving! Now, if we divide 108 fat calories by the 180 total calories, we find that the "reduced fat" peanut butter is made up of a whopping 60 percent fat! (See label next page.)

Reduced-fat? Yes. Reduced enough? We say no way! But hey, we eat what we want. We just don't trust everything we read.

How does this compare to the regular stuff? Regular peanut butter has 200 calories and 16 grams of fat in the same two tablespoons. That calculates to 72 percent fat!

This is just an example of how you can eat what you want, but in a logical way. Remember, a two tablespoon serving of reduced-fat peanut butter gets 60 percent of its calories from fat! So much for that "reduced-fat" label. But, guess what? You can still have that peanut butter. Mel does quite often: "I frequently have difficulty getting enough protein at my breakfast meal. Like this morning, I knew I needed at least 400 calories before I went for my activity break. Breakfast was one and one half whole wheat English muffins, ONE half of one

Nutrition Facts

Serving Size 2 Tbsp. (35g)

Servings Per Container 14

Amount Per Serving

Calories 180   Calories From Fat 100

% Daily Value*

Total Fat 12g	**19%**
Saturated Fat 2.5g	**12%**
Sodium 170 mg	**7%**
Total Carbohydrate 13g	**4%**
Sugars 4g	
Protein 8g	
Calcium 0%	Magnesium 15%
Dietary Fiber 2g	

*Percent Daily Values are based on a 2,000 calorie diet. Your daily values may be higher or lower depending on your calorie needs:

	Calories	2,000	2,500
Total Fat	Less than	65g	80g
Sat Fat	Less than	20g	25g
Cholesterol	Less than	300mg	300mg
Sodium	Less than	2,400mg	2,400mg
Total Carbohydrate		300g	375g
Dietary Fiber	25g	30g	

Nutrition label from a jar of "reduced-fat" peanut butter

muffin had one and one half teaspoons of peanut butter. Yes, I could see it on there. I could feel it and smell it too! It tasted wonderful. It really is adequate! This means I only ate one-fourth the standard serving, so the total fat grams were only three. Yes, the percentage stayed the same. But, on the other two halves of muffins I put some nonfat cream cheese and some low-fat turkey breast, about a half an ounce each. I also had a banana. When the meal was built, it was about 9 percent calories from fat."

Here's another example. This one is an organic vegetarian burrito that really tastes great, by the way!

Is this one a gold mine or what? One fat gram times 9 calories per gram equals 9 fat calories. Now, divide by 260 and you get only 3 percent of the calories from fat! And look at all the protein and complex carbos! Not to mention all of that fiber. You don't do much better than 7 grams per serving. If you see any label with this kind of profile, you are guaranteed to get a nutritious meal.

Nutrition Facts
Nutrition Facts
Serving size: 1 burrito (168g)
Servings per container: 1
Amount per serving
Calories 260   Calories From Fat 10

Nutrition Facts

Serving size: 1 burrito (168g)

Servings per container: 1

Amount per serving

Calories 260   Calories From Fat 10

	% Daily Value*
Total Fat 1g	**2%**
Saturated Fat 0g	**0%**
Sodium 490 mg	**20%**
Total Carbohydrate 48g	**18%**
Sugars 2g	
Protein 13g	
Calcium 10%	Iron 15%
Vitamin A 10%	Vitamin C 25%
Fiber 7 gm	

*Percent Daily Values are based on a 2,000 calorie diet. Your daily values may be higher or lower depending on your calorie needs:

	Calories	2,000	2,500
Total Fat	Less than	65g	80g
Sat Fat	Less than	20g	25g
Cholesterol	Less than	300mg	300mg
Sodium	Less than	2,400mg	2,400mg
Total Carbohydrate		300g	375g
Dietary Fiber		25g	30g

Nutrition label from an organically-grown vegetarian burrito

We doctor up this "fast food." It only takes a couple of minutes in the microwave. About thirty seconds before it is finished cooking, toss on an extra ounce or two of fat-free or low-fat cheese, then finish it off. Top with some fat-free sour cream and a ton of salsa and it's Mexican to the max!

Let's try some math on a candy bar. Two and one-half grams of fat times 9 calories per gram equals 22½ calories from fat. If we divide the number of fat calories by the total number of calories in the candy bar we find that 32 percent of its calories come from fat! And this candy bar is only about the size of a Halloween candy bar! Think what a full-sized one contains!

Nutrition Facts

Serving Size 1 bar (20 g)
Servings Per Container 9

Amount Per Serving
Calories 70   Calories From Fat 25

	% DailyValue*
Total Fat 2.5g	**4%**
Saturated Fat 1g	**5%**
Sodium 75 mg	**3%**
Total Carbohydrate 12g	**4%**
Sugars 9g	
Protein 1g	
Calcium 2%	

Not a significant source of cholesterol, dietary fiber, vitamin A, vitamin C, and iron.

*Percent Daily Values are based on a 2,000 calorie diet. Your daily values may be higher or lower depending on your calorie needs:

	Calories	2,000	2,500
Total Fat	Less than	65g	80g
Sat Fat	Less than	20g	25g
Cholesterol	Less than	300mg	300mg
Sodium	Less than	2,400mg	2,400mg
Total Carbohydrate		300g	375g
Dietary Fiber		25g	30g

Nutrition label from a small candy bar

How about this one?

A soft bagel, plain. It has 210 calories and contains 1 gram of fat.
You try the calculation: Fat grams = _____ x _____ = _____
divided by _____ = _____% calories from fat.

Try this one, too!
Ready-to-eat, high-fiber cereal, a ½ cup serving has 60 calories

and contains 1 gram of fat. Fat grams = _____ x _____ = _____ divided by _____ = _____% calories from fat!

Having trouble with the math? You know what we are going to do? We have placed our phone number and address in the resource section of the book. If you can't get the math, either in this chapter or other ones, all you have to do is ask for help. If a bit of math or some other question means the difference between successfully changing your life for the better versus giving up before you start, we are more than happy to help. Another frustration with other so-called diet books, is there is no one to contact if you have questions. You can contact us. That's part of BodyLogic

Now go defat that kitchen. Start by tossing (or donating) anything with more than 3 fat grams per serving. Be sure and keep at least one of your favorite PMS foods, or the one thing that if you had to do without in its present state, you would feel deprived. It must be the one food that brings you more pleasure than any other, and for which there is no tolerable substitute.

Now go through what's left in your kitchen and practice fat percentage calculations. You will be amazed at where the fat is hidden.

Your goal should be to keep your fat intake between 10 and 30 percent of calories from fat. You can calculate this a number of ways. The easiest for most people is not to put anything in your mouth that is greater than 10–30 percent calories from fat, whichever number you select is your choice and based on how your body reacts. Consuming a high-fiber diet will help remove some of the deposits of fat in your arteries, plus it will help keep you regular. It will fill you up and keep you fuller longer. Fat has a wonderful lubricating effect and you may notice some initial problems with constipation. But moving your body, drinking plenty of water and increasing the fiber in your diet will keep the digestive tract functioning just fine.

Another way of tracking fat is to determine your total fat percentage allotment for the day and keep track as the day goes. We find this rather obsessive/compulsive, but sometimes it is helpful while you are learning what the fat content is in various foods. Example: Mel's recommended daily intake of calories based on height, weight and activity level is 2,200–2,600 calories per day. She prefers a diet of 10 percent calories from fat. That's easy enough to calculate: 22–26 grams per day. She can keep track as the day goes, or she can divide those grams up between her various meals, but again you may be like Mel and find this too constrictive. Most of us like flexibility and choice. If you want to go out to brunch and have real scrambled eggs, you will soon know two eggs takes 14 of your fat grams for the day—leaves the rest of the day fairly restricted, but that's one choice you can make. Managing your food plan like this does not mean that you don't eat the next day just because you exceeded your fat gram count the day before. Just eat more quality food to replace the fat calories for that one day! Look at your food intake around mid afternoon. Where do you stand with your percentages? If you are too low on fat, plan on some peanut butter and an apple for a snack, or you might choose low-fat cottage cheese or low-fat frozen yogurt instead of the fat-free variety. You may just eat your usual low-fat or fat-free fare and plan to increase your fat a bit the next day. You don't have to live by numbers and keep the calculator with you wherever you go. In time, you will be able to review your day's foodstyle in your head and know if your diet is balanced. If you are like us, you may not eat many vegetables in the morning and at noon, so we always have three or four servings for the evening meal. That's not hard to do with a huge Caesar salad and some frozen, mixed veggies.

So now decide on the fat percentage that you want to start with. If you are accustomed to a high-fat diet, start at 30–40 percent of calories from fat and gradually work down. Go back through that kitchen and toss or donate anything greater than your fat percentage. For example, if you plan to start at 20 percent calories from fat, get rid of anything that has more than 20 percent calories from fat per serving. Still keep that one favorite food though! Hang onto most of your quality beef, poultry and fish. Fat percentages may not be known and it does not matter. We will show you later how you can modify your recipes to get the total fat percentage per serving down to a level with which you are happy.

If you learn nothing else, remember this: There are good fats and bad fats. Good fats are those liquid at room temperature, like olive oil, peanut oil, canola oil. Bad fats are more solid at room temperature, like coconut oil and animal fats. You find coconut or palm oil in chocolate. That's what makes the candy bar hard rather than gooey. Imagine what that does to your arteries! Also remember this: Whether "good" or "bad" fat, fat is still fat. Look at labels. Let's take "light" margarine for example. It may have fewer fat grams per serving, but it is still 100 percent calories from fat! Yes, a step in the right direction, but you can do much better. Jan learned this lesson when she went food shopping with Mel one weekend. "And I thought I was doing so well by using the lighter version. I didn't realize it was still 100 percent fat. The food labels really do seem to lie, unless you know how to make sense of them." Shortening and olive oil both contain 100 percent calories from fat. Fat is still fat. No matter what the form!

Let's go shopping!

Now make up a shopping list of those items you can't do without as well as those items you could eliminate, but don't want to if you could find some healthier substitutions. Fortunately these days, there is a lower-fat or fat-free version for most everything. Looks can be deceiving, so when you go to the store, look forward to some strangers staring at you while you pull out your calculator. Actually, we discovered many others doing the very same thing! Mel has even found herself conducting impromptu classes in the middle of the grocery store when fascinated onlookers start asking questions and become totally intrigued with the concept! Do not confuse "percent of daily fat" written on the label with "percent of calories from fat" per serving. There is a huge difference. Select versions of those foods on your list that are within your desired fat percentage per serving. (We have provided a list of substitutions in the reference chapter, just to save you a bit of time!) While you are at it, experiment with a few new foods you have never tried before that sound good. Variety is the spice of life! Over the next few weeks, go through your spice cabinet and replace anything that is a year or more old. Flavors die. This stuff doesn't stay good forever. One secret to cutting the fat is to replace the fat with other flavors, not to mention moisture and texture. The first few trips to the store will be long ones. Don't forget to eat before you go. *Never go grocery shopping when the gas tank is empty!* (This means the gas tank in the car, as well as the one in your body!)

It's all about balance. It's not so much what you do day to day, but how the numbers average out over time. If you want to go out for pizza, go for it. Have a couple slices of veggie cheese pizza (hold the meat). That's a fairly healthy meal. Just cut back the fat a bit over the next couple of days, maybe by 3 or 4 grams/day. Things will average out. What's important is that you stick to a routine percentage of calories from fat on most days.

In time, all of this number crunching and obsession over fat grams will no longer be necessary. Your new eating patterns will be just as automatic as your old ones were! You will learn what brands to buy and automatically reach for them, rather than the higher fat varieties. You will laugh when you continue to search for *low-fat peanut butter*! It isn't out there yet, folks! Check out the diet food section, which you will notice is becoming nearly nonexistent in most stores. Look at the jar of the so-called diet peanut butter. It says in very small print "Not a low-calorie food," yet the label might say something like "50 percent less sugar than regular varieties." Look at the fat grams: 14 GRAMS PER SERVING! This stuff belongs on the shelf with the rest of the peanut butter. Not to mention the fact that you are probably spending much more for it than you should have to, just because it is in a specialty section. What a joke!

Mel candidly discusses her favorite topic: food fraud!

Some days I find grocery shopping and eating out experiences that anger me and insult my intelligence. I try to do some positive thinking and find some entertainment in identifying "FOOD FRAUD," then coming up with a way to help reverse that trend. Enjoy being a strong enough person to refuse food that insults your body! Feel free to have just a beverage. If you are hungry but nothing on the menu is consistent with your food choices, and the cook will not fill a special request, politely thank the waitperson then get up and leave. You can do better. Your body deserves it. Smile as the employees watch you go into the establishment across the street, and not come out for an hour or so! I mean really, any cook who will not fix my omelet with egg whites or egg substitute in this day and age isn't worth my time, money or most impor-tantly my health! Ask questions. Be leery of those little red hearts next to certain menu items, those professing to be healthier choices. So what is healthier? Maybe the fact that you get a smaller serving than what is on the regular menu? So starvation is healthy? We know better. I once was traveling to the beach and stopped for lunch at a typical coffee-shop type place. I look through the "healthy" menu and spot a turkey sandwich on twelve-grain bread.

Sounds pretty good to me! Comes with green salad, too! When the waitperson came, I asked what all came on the sandwich. She replied, "Turkey, lettuce, sprouts, and mayo." I said, "Excuse me, did you say mayo? Is that fat-free or low-fat mayo?" She replied, "No ma'am, just regular mayo." I was willing to give her the benefit of the doubt on that one, and politely asked to have her substitute mustard (Dijon if possible) on the side. No problem. So far so good. She asked what kind of dressing I would like on the salad. Of course I asked what kind they had and she rattled off a list of fatty, oily stuff. I asked if she had any low-cal or nonfat dressing. She said, "I'm sorry ma'am but we don't. I could bring you some vinegar or lemon juice." Now I'm beginning to wonder. "I'll think about it for a minute. What else comes with the meal?" She said, "French fries, no substitutions." At that point I blew a gasket. Now anyone who knows me knows it takes a lot to pull my chain, but this was the last straw. I not so nicely, and in a loud enough voice for all to hear, proceeded to explain the concept of "healthy cuisine" in a manner that I will not repeat here. Needless to say, I refuse to pay full price for a meal, if I choose not to eat half or have half of the food left off the plate because the restaurant won't substitute items and then not be able to enjoy my food! Who wants a dry sandwich, dry or bitter lettuce and nothing else when it's four hours till the next stop? Worse yet, who wants to eat what others force you to eat knowing you will feel sick later? I said my piece and promptly got up and left. I found a much more accommodating establishment just down the street. And you know what? I was proud of myself. I knew that day that my lifestyle had changed for the better, and I would never fall back into my old lifestyle again. I had grown my inside, and shrank my outside, and had acquired a new found sense of self-confidence that I did not know was a part of me. I knew I was in control for once in my life! Now, when I go out to eat and see some obviously healthy selections, I play games once in a while, quiz the waitperson extensively, and select an item with lots of potential for substitutions and see what happens. If it's no problem, I come back!

Go out to eat and have fun. Go to your typical breakfast place. Order a veggie cheese omelet that comes with hash browns and toast, and say the following: "I'll have the veggie cheese omelet with egg substitute or egg white only, put just enough cheese on it so I can see it and no more, throw in a few extra veggies and please sauté those dry, without oil or butter, before they go inside the omelet. Hold the hash browns and substitute a bowl of oatmeal, no butter, no sugar and hold the cream."

When you live this way, you can have your cake and eat it too! (Literally!) No deprivation allowed! One final note. Everything we discuss in this book will become habit over time. Once these concepts become habit, you will have changed your lifestyle. Because you will be feeling so good, the likelihood of reverting back to your old ways is slim to none, excuse the pun!

You are not dieting. You are providing your body with high-octane fuel so you will feel better and live longer. Eat when you are hungry, but only until you are full. Make sure you eat enough!

The only thing you CAN'T have is the food you say you CAN'T have! There is no such thing in your life as can't have when it comes to food. It's what you choose to have or not to have. That's BodyLogic!

Here's an update on Jan. "I am sleeping less. I am now rested after only six hours of sleep at night. A few months ago, I needed nine to ten hours of sleep per night to make it through my work day. My, what a difference in such a short amount of time!"

> ***Your positive self statement for today: I am living for the present. I am making changes to guide my future.***

Overdue for a Lube Job and Oil Change?

The FatLogic of BodyLogic

The greatest gift you can give yourself is the gift of health. You can be overfat and improve your health at the same time!

Let's recap for a moment. You have taken a good hard look at your childhood, your life today, and your relationship with food. You may not have uncovered all of the details yet, but that's OK. You now know what your body *needs* with regard to calories in order to get adequate nutrition. You know how to find fat in your food. You have defatted your kitchen and have decided on a fat level that is correct for you, somewhere between 10 and 30 percent calories from fat. Your immediate goal is *not* to lose weight, but to feel better and healthier. You have made excellent progress so far. Before you can move on to the next level of BodyLogic, it is time to start loving yourself and your body, just as you are today!

You will find no humor in this chapter, because this is one of the most serious topics. You must be clear in your own mind as to what you can reasonably expect from BodyLogic. BodyLogic works only if *you* work on healing your mind as well as your body. To focus on the body and not the mind means you are on yet another "diet" and we're sorry to say you are destined to fail before you have begun.

Before you can move forward, you must make the commitment to change your life forever. Though today it may seem daunting, in time it will be nearly effortless. FatLogic will be the hardest thing for you to deal with on a daily basis, and you will deal with that for the rest of your life.

What is FatLogic? FatLogic is accepting yourself for who you are, and realizing that it is not so much what people see on the outside that puts you in a "fat" category. It is how you feel about yourself on the inside that makes you a "fat" person in the eyes of yourself and those around you. If you are truly committed to making a lifelong change that will give you more pleasure and pride than anything else you have ever experienced or had in material things, please say the following affirmation, out loud, to yourself, in front of a mirror:

I (state your name) love myself. I am worthy of everything wonderful in life, including food. I am a good person. Eating food does not make me good or bad. Food is my fuel. The larger my body, and the more I move my body, the more fuel my body needs. From this day forward, I will treat my body as the very special, one-of-a-kind life form that it was created to be. I will start and end each day in a healthy way, but will not speak ill of myself if I am not "perfect" in-between, because I am human, and no one is perfect. I will no longer fear food. Instead, I will give it the same level of respect that I give the air that I breathe, and the water that I drink. Without food, my body would die. Food is necessary for my physical life. It is not necessary for my psyche. Food will no longer be a substitute for love, safety, or any other feeling that I am lacking emotionally.

I vow never, ever to diet again because starvation destroys living things. I vow to look in the mirror and make at least one positive statement about my body each day. I vow to try to avoid negative self-talk. I vow to be a strong person and stand up for what is important to me. I will not let others rule my life or my food. I will not become obsessed with counting calories or grams of anything. I vow to destroy my scale and never purchase another. I will never fear food again!

I will move my body within my comfort zone. I will eat when hungry, eat what I like, and eat the best fuel I can give my body whenever possible, because I am ready to change my life forever.

I (state your name) love myself. I don't care what others think of me. I am beautiful in my present state. If I choose to set goals for myself with regard to fat loss or activity, I vow that they will be realistic ones. I vow to stop trying to kill myself in order to be like someone whom I can never be. My outside body may be large, but it is my psyche that makes me a fat person. No matter what size the outside of my body is, I will still be a fat person in my soul, and that is a wonderful thing. I will be myself, because that is the best I can be.

Now, say that to yourself again several times. Write it down in a letter to yourself and put copies of that letter on your bathroom mirror, your refrigerator, in your panty drawer, wherever you will be forced to see it on a daily basis, and say it on a daily basis. Look in the mirror as you say it. Make a mental note of the person you are today, both physically and emotionally. Don't ever forget what it feels like to be who you are *today*. This will be a reference point for you in the future. If you are so inclined, start a daily diary, not just a food diary. Begin writing the story of your new life which starts today. As you shed fat, you will need smaller clothing sizes. Save one of your largest size pair of pants (preferably not elastic waisted), one blouse and one dress. The first time you drop a size, wrap up the selected clothing in a box, gift wrap it, and stick it away in the closet with a card that reads something like: "To_____(enter your name). The best gift I ever gave myself." When the time comes for you to move into maintenance with BodyLogic, then give yourself a birth-day party. The gift you stashed away can then be opened. Try on those clothes and take some pictures of yourself. Mel did this in private with a timer on her camera. It is a very special moment, best enjoyed in the pleasure of your own company.

Mel has one regret about changing her lifestyle:

I did not keep a diary along the way. I recognize that I have grown spiritually and that spiritual growth never stops. I consider this change in lifestyle to be the greatest gift I ever gave myself, and I pray that I never lose sight of the person I was before, because I don't want to be that exact same woman ever again.

A large part of me has not changed. The one thing I find the most amazing is how I still see myself as and consider myself to be a fat person. For example, I bought a new fanny pack which was too big, even when I cinched the straps up as tight as they would go. I did not consider trying it on in the middle of the isle before I bought it. I now recognize yet another part of that fat person which still remains, fear of having someone else see me try some-thing on that does not fit. I still saw a 220-pound plus person in the mirror as I struggled with adjusting those straps. Though my clothing sizes are much smaller, I still somewhat hate going clothes shopping, for the fear I won't find anything I like that fits! I now wear Petite sizes, which in a way I hate because once again I am placed in a size category. I have always been sensitive about my weight and my size. I hated being fitted for band uniforms because my size was never available. I was squished into someone else's size, so tight that I was afraid to bend over for fear of splitting out the seat of my pants. So tight that every lump and bulge showed. So tight that the sleeves of the tops would only go half way as far up my arms as they should go, making for a most uncomfortable fit and unpleasant sight. It was the same way with gym and girl scout uniforms. My first recollection comes from age six, going school clothes shopping and stopping to reach for a beautiful top. My mother said, "That won't fit you. We have to go the 'Chubby Department.'" God, I hated that word "chubby." You see, as a small child, before I had fully begun to see myself as different from the other children, society was teaching me that I was different, and in a negative way. Even during my high school senior photos, they had to find an extension to secure the feather wrap around my shoulders and chest. The back gaped open. I was soooo embarrassed.

My new size certainly is not associated with the same negativism as a "Plus Size" department (at least in my mind), but a category none the less. The selection is still limited, and the prices are higher than in the regular Misses section. I still don't own a swimsuit, and would not comfortably wear shorts in public until this last summer. Yes, I have a lot of growing yet to do. I will always be a fat person on the inside. I always have been. That is the only me I know. But that old me has come a long way from hiding behind food to confronting issues head on. Instead of using my fat psyche as a protective shield, I now use it as my source of strength and power with which to move forward and explore new things, and stand up for myself when the going gets tough rather than retreating into solitary confinement with a bag of potato chips.

In trying to come up with a title for this book, we received several suggestions. Some really struck a very sensitive spot in my heart—how it feels to be fat. I always have been overly sensitive about my weight. I hated being put into the "fat" category, and my heart still sinks any time I see such references made about overfat people. The worst for me today is to see one or several children teasing another child who is overfat, and looking at the expression on that child's face. It makes me want to cry, and often I do.

Being fat is similar to being an alcoholic. You can kick the habit, but you still remain an alcoholic. You can quit using food as a substitute for love and safety, but you will always be fat on the inside. We think that's a good thing. What better strength to keep you moving ahead! What better motivation to continue on your path of healing?

We say these things to you in an effort to give you hope, to help you feel good about yourself no matter what your body looks like, and most importantly to let you know that a smaller physical body will not change anything in your psyche. It is up to you to change that. A smaller body will not make you more popular, it will not bring you wealth, it in and of itself will not bring you total happiness. It is the growth you experience as a part of the process, and the continued growth you experience in maintaining that new lifestyle, that changes the psyche and makes you happier. This happiness and self-confidence will be what draws other people to you. When you grow the inside, body changes will follow!

You have made a serious commitment to yourself to change. That is by far the hardest part of BodyLogic. We did not give that to you. You found it within yourself. Be elated with having completed level one. Celebrate! This is the first day of your new life! Make note of this day on your calendar, and in your diary. Spend the rest of this day celebrating yourself! Get your hair colored! Pamper yourself! Turn to the recipe chapter and make up a batch of extra special fudge brownies, to eat the next time you are hungry of course! Love yourself!

Your positive self statement for today: I Love Myself! Love of myself, love of my body. My eyes are my mirror, they tell the story.

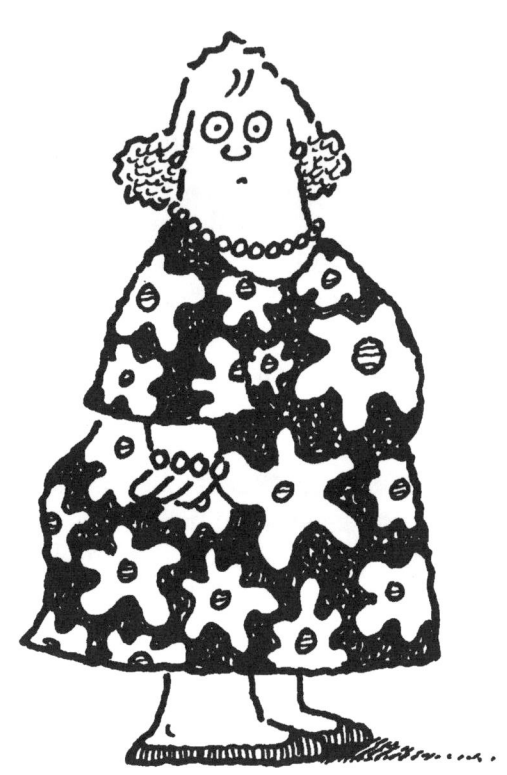

Computerized Diagnostics

FoodLogic, Step by Step

The Pyramid

Remember what we said before: It's not the quantity of the food, but the quality of the food that counts. It's not the portions, it's the proportions. In order for BodyLogic to work, you must change your attitude about food. Food is your friend. Good food will not make your body fat. Good food increases metabolism which in turn burns more fat. Fat will make your body fat. Fat slows down the rate that food can be used by your body. Food is a basic need. Good fuel is high-octane gas for your engine. Good food helps repair the damage from dieting. Skipping meals makes you fat. Not eating makes you fat, fat and more fat (or dead)!

From here on out, always think about food in terms of what you need, not what you can or cannot have. That is the hardest thing to overcome, the fear of food. If you are like us, you will fight the battle of "food fear" for the rest of your life. Please give yourself permission to eat what you need, eat what you want, and eat what you like, as long as you use your logic and not your emotions in making those choices. It's that simple. That's BodyLogic! That's FoodLogic! That's good old-fashioned common sense! You can eat your way into a new and improved body, and enjoy every minute of it.

Before we get into this chapter, we want to forewarn you, some of the concepts may again seem overwhelming. They may be too structured for you. If that is the case, please do not put the book down and say "I'll never get all of this!" You don't have to get all of it all at once. Remember, one small step at a time. Don't try to completely change everything about your foodstyle all at once. Start with reducing the fat. That is the most important. Then advance to reducing refined sugar. From there, you can start incorporating more defined meal planning if you want to. Remember, we are not asking you to eat as we do. We are giving you the tools to plan your own Body-Logic lifestyle change. Think of it this way. Let's pretend your foodstyle change is like a tool box. The tool box contains many different tools. You may choose to use only one or a few of them. That's fine. When you tighten a loose screw on a cabinet door, and pull out the tool box, do you use every tool in that box to repair the cabinet door? Likely not. It's the same way with FoodLogic. Use what you need, when you need it, and in a way that is comfortable for you.

If you choose to incorporate just some of the concepts, we encourage you to focus on the fats. In the reference chapter we have included a food substitutions/shopping list. It is titled "Health Foods." Tear it out and keep it in your handbag, so the next time you go to the store, you will have part of your tool box with you! We have done much of the work for you. Make your foodstyle change an adventure in addition to a learning experience. Make it a labor of love for yourself. Please do not make it weigh too heavily on your shoulders. If you do, it will be difficult to slowly incorporate the changes needed to be healthy for life. Play investigator when you go shopping. We are not perfect, and neither are you. Just do the best you can and that will be good enough! That's what Melonie's father always told her. It was one of the most loving things he ever said, and he said it often. Say it to yourself at least once a day!

Let's begin with a brief lesson in biochemistry. We will make it as light as possible. The purpose is to teach you how the body uses and reacts to the various types of fuel it is given. Think again of your car. Have you ever heard a car knocking? Especially an older car? One reason it knocks is because the fuel it has in its tank is not high enough quality to keep its engine running smoothly. When you move your body and feel pain, or see stuff jiggle, or get out of breath, visualize and listen for that "knocking" engine. Here's an example for you computer nerds out there. Does your computer ever slow down or freeze up after you have been using it for a long time, especially opening and closing numerous programs or running several programs at the same time? The computer acts this way because its memory is fragmented. Rebooting that computer will defragment that old RAM, and things will once again run smoothly for a while. You can buy a software program that takes care of the problem as it happens, before you notice it. Your body works the same way. If it does not have enough power, or if it is being abused by poor fueling and lack of activity, it functions in a fragmented way. Quality fuel and activity gives it the power it needs to function smoothly, and prevent it from "freezing up" on you!

Here's one we think almost everyone can relate to. You have a houseplant that has been doing OK for years, and all of a sudden its leaves drop, it droops, and it looks like it's going to kick the bucket. No matter how much or how little water you give it, it doesn't get better. You re-pot the thing. It's still sick. Just when you have about given up, it dawns on you that the poor thing has not had a good shot of fertilizer for a long time. You feed the plant, and it grows! You get rid of the old branches and dead leaves (the dead weight) and it thrives! BodyLogic works the same way. Years of starving your body of what it needs causes it to drop, droop and look like it's going to kick the bucket! Fertilize your body regularly and reduce some of the dead weight that drains the life-sustaining resources, and it will "blossom" before your very eyes.

Let's focus now on your body, and what types of fuel it needs to thrive and be strong.

Protein, the building blocks of life!

Proportionately, your body needs about half as much protein as it does carbohydrate, which is a pretty amazing fact. Protein is essential to build muscle and tissues. The more you move your body, the more lifting you do, the more protein you need. Did you know that for every day of bed rest, like when you are sick with the flu, you can lose as much as 3–5 percent of your muscle mass? When you are not eating enough and not moving enough, you lose muscle. Muscle is your ticket to fat burning. Muscle provides the strength to move your body around. Muscle is what makes you look toned and healthy. Protein is necessary to build the basic structure of every cell, including the cells that make up muscle tissue. Protein is required to help enzymes and hormones work. It is found in nearly every part of your body, including your skin, muscle, bones, teeth and blood. Unless you eat sufficient calories to meet your metabolic needs, your body may not get enough protein. If you don't eat enough quality food, your body will use the muscle and other tissue it has from which to obtain its protein. Cannibalism! Too much protein in your diet is not harmful as a rule unless you are using protein calories to replace carbohydrate calories. If this is the case, your body does not have enough complex carbohydrate to supply its energy needs. Your body will attempt to use fat before protein for energy. There are several so-called diets out there that make you survive on a ridiculously low amount of carbohydrate, and force protein down your throat. We tried them. We felt awful. We did lose weight, but we did not lose fat. There came a point where we both experienced such fatigue and carbohydrate cravings that we gave in. We instantly felt better, threw away those diet books, and gained every bit of that weight back. The problem was, the weight gain was fat and water, not muscle. Muscle requires good fuel plus stress (e.g. exercise) in order to grow strong and stay strong. Read on to learn why.

Complex carbohydrates—gas for the engine!

Complex carbos are your body's most immediate and efficient fuel source. Unfortunately, unlike fat and protein, carbohydrates cannot be stored for use later. Instead, if there is an excess, they are con-verted to fat which of course is stored as fat. The body must have a regular supply of carbohydrate in order to meet its energy needs. They break down into glucose which feeds the brain. Your body needs a lot of this kind of fuel to function optimally. Think of it this way. What tends to give you better gas mileage in your car, regular unleaded or super unleaded? Which fuel tends to make your car run more smoothly? Unless you own a car designed to function best on the lower grade, you likely would notice a difference. Here is an-other example. Your car breaks down on a stormy night, and you decide to camp out. You are very cold and decide to start a campfire. You find dry wood, but you have no matches. You remember hear-ing that you can rub two stones or two sticks together to make a spark to start your fire. After you have tried this method for a couple of hours, you remember that emergency matchbook in your glove box. In ten seconds, you have a warming fire.

Your body works the same way. Think of simple carbohydrates (like refined sugar, white sugar, brown sugar, white flour and starchy things which break down into simple sugars) as lower octane gas, or two cold stones or a damp pair of sticks. Think of complex carbohydrates as premium, high octane gas or a dry book of matches. Complex carbos get your metabolism burning quickly. They are the fuel for your fire! Good sources of complex carbos are whole grains, beans, legumes, and most fresh fruits and vegetables. And don't forget the nutritional punch that complex carbos provide: vitamins, minerals, trace elements and protein. Eat enough of these, and you won't need to pad the pockets of vitamin manufacturers. Interestingly, these foods are most often found in their natural state. Why mess with Mother Nature?

So what happens if you restrict carbos? As hinted at above in the protein section, the body breaks down fat to use as fuel. You may think, isn't that what we want? In this instance, the body is forced to break down more fat than what it was designed to handle. It has to work too hard at it. There is an accumulation of acids in the body which are by-products of the fat breakdown process. This is called acidosis. As a defense mechanism, the body attaches salt (sodium) to these acids so they can be excreted in the urine. This can result in severe sodium depletion and electrolyte imbalance. Electrolyte imbalance can cause dehydration, diarrhea, kidney problems, heart problems, coma and even death.

Carbohydrates function in the liver and other organs to convert bacteria, metabolic by-products and other toxins so they can be excreted. Carbohydrates are essential for healthy nerve and brain tissue. A constant supply of complex carbohydrate keeps the blood sugar on an even keel, unlike the response to simple or refined carbohydrates.

Simple carbohydrates cause dramatic swings in blood sugar. Eating these foods triggers the pancreas to increase secretion of insulin. Insulin converts the sugar into a form that can be used to provide energy to the muscles, storage of glycogen (like an energy reserve) in the liver, and increasing the uptake of glucose by fat to be converted to fat and stored for later use. The problem is, it doesn't take as long to break down simple carbos as it does complex carbos. Therefore, when the simple carbos have been broken down, a fairly high level of insulin remains in the blood stream. Now the blood sugar is low, which triggers the brain to send out hunger signals, even though you just ate something. Looking at it from a different standpoint, if you consume complex carbos, they take longer to be broken down. By the time these foods have been broken down, insulin levels are no longer high. They are falling off back toward normal levels. The brain says, "blood sugar is about right for insulin level, so I guess the body is fine for now. No food needed."

Simply stated, you feel fuller, longer after eating complex carbos than after eating simple carbos. If you have ever missed lunch and grabbed a candy bar to tide you over, have you ever noticed how sleepy you became within an hour or so after eating? Did you notice how hungry you felt? Did it trigger the urge to grab a second candy bar, some chips or a cookie? And did this keep going until you finally got a decent meal into your stomach? In the case of a diabetic, their pancreas is not able to produce enough insulin. Without enough insulin, carbos do not get broken down, so they cannot be used for energy. Instead, they are dumped in the urine. In a way, diabetes causes the body to starve. When diabetics take too much insulin, their blood sugar drops too low, and they can end up in acidosis, which can progress rapidly to coma and death.

Really watch those food labels. Fat-free does not necessarily mean healthy complex carbos. Avoid products loaded with refined sugar. Try to find cold cereals that are made from whole grains, are high in protein and fiber, and have no added sugar. Another thing with cold cereals, when you read the labels watch the serving sizes. Some will have as many as 200 calories per half cup serving! Who eats just a half cup? Won't satisfy you very much most likely!

Fats, can't live with 'em, can't live without 'em!

As mentioned before, fats are the most concentrated energy source, providing 9 calories per gram. You have probably noticed that oil and water do not mix. The body contains a huge amount of water which is necessary for the utilization of protein and carbohydrates. These substances do mix with water. Blood contains water. There-fore, these are more easily distributed to the body. Because fat is not easily dissolved in water, it is used as our body's "mini-storage" if you will. Any extra carbohydrate, or protein that we eat which our body does not need at the time is converted to fat and stored for later use. The majority of the fats we eat are also stored. This is the body's defense mechanism to prevent death during starvation. Think again of the bear hibernating. If the bear's body did not have fat to fall back on, the bear would die in his sleep! Fat is the body's potato cellar, the grain silo, the food bank. Up to two thirds of the total energy of our cells may be supplied by our fat stores rather than by carbohydrate.

Fats add a lot more than what we see on the outside of our bodies. Fats slow down the emptying time of the stomach, making us feel fuller longer. Certain vitamins do not dissolve in water. They require fat as their vehicle to be transported to the various parts of the body. Fat or adipose tissue keeps the body warm and protects the organs and nerves. Fat also makes food taste better. Fat is what gives foods that smooth, creamy, rich texture. We need to eat some fat every day. Fats contain essential fatty acids which play important roles in the transport and metabolism of fat and maintain the function of cells. They can also lower cholesterol. The problem is, essential fatty acids are not stored, nor can they be manufactured by the body. Essential fatty acids are found in vegetable oils, like canola or olive oil. They are also found in nuts and poultry. Fats should be consumed sparingly, and chosen from those sources that contain essential fatty acids. Your body only needs a small amount of essential fatty acids each day, and this quantity can easily be supplied by a well-balanced food intake without having to add any extra fat.

The fats you eat should be mono- or polyunsaturated. These are the good fats that provide essential fatty acids and help to lower cholesterol. Saturated fats and hydrogenated fats should be avoided whenever possible. These are the ones that clog your arteries! Food labels will give you the quantities of the different kinds of fats. Choose products that are higher in mono- and polyunsaturated fats than saturated fat. As a rule of thumb, hydrogenated and saturated fats retain their shape at room temperature, and become firm or hard in the fridge. Think of stick butter, shortening and stick margarine. Also think of what fat on a steak looks like. These are saturated and hydrogenated fats. Choose well-trimmed, extra-lean cuts of meat. All fats are not created equal! Just remember, fat is fat. What isn't used by the body is stored as fat. It's that simple.

This is a very simplistic overview of the role of carbohydrates, proteins and fat. The purpose is not to give you a graduate degree in biochemistry, but to help you understand why each of these nutrients are so important, and that they be consumed in the right proportions. If a little is good, a lot is not better in this case! That's Body-Logic. Give the body just what it needs, when it needs it, and it will take care of the rest. Give the body just enough fat to supply essential fatty acids, give the body a constant, but not excessive supply of carbohydrate, and give the body an adequate supply of protein. This way, when extra fuel is needed, fat is broken down for energy, while protein stays in the tissues and bones where it needs to be to provide strength.

Doing this results in a slow rate of fat loss over time. This fat loss is the kind of weight loss you want. This is one area in which we agree with the experts. Slower weight loss over time is more apt to result in permanent weight management. The only kind of weight loss that occurs slowly is fat loss. Lets say you did not drink any fluids for a day. (We don't recommend this!) If you weighed yourself the next morning, you likely would have lost several pounds of weight—water weight that is. As soon as you replaced the fluids you lost through various body processes, that weight loss would be a thing of the past. If you don't eat enough protein, your body will use what it has stored. This process does not take very long. Rapid weight loss can be a reflection of muscle loss. Why do you want to lose something so important?

Remember, breakdown of carbohydrate and protein is twice as fast as fat. Calories are simply the amount of energy or heat produced when a quantity of food is broken down. To repeat, carbohydrate and protein each contain 4 calories per gram. Fat contains 9 calories per gram. Fat gives off more energy when broken down because it takes longer to break down—twice as long! So, when you lose muscle instead of fat, the rate of "weight" loss is faster.

If "fat" loss is your goal, please be elated for as slow a rate of loss as possible. This means your body is keeping what it needs, and getting rid of the rest. Think of your body's "fat" loss as its garage sale! If you lose "weight" too quickly, you are probably getting rid of something that you will later regret, like muscle! Drink lots of water. Don't feel like you are drowning, but you should try to get eight cups a day. Water helps to metabolize fat. Water is also lost when you exercise.

So you see, it's not the portion size that counts so much as the proportions, the ratios of carbs to protein to fats. First carbs, which you need the most of. Proteins come second. You know what comes last, that which you likely already have too much of—fat! Quantity of food is not so important if you eat when you are really hungry, and eat in a balanced way!

Calculating the miles per gallon

For as many textbooks and diet books as there are available, there are at least as many opinions regarding which percentages of calories from protein, carbohydrate and fat you should consume. Our experience has been that the percentages quoted in medical textbooks are often for "normal" people. BodyLogic works for the rest of us, people who have been carrying around a lot of extra fat for a long time. Most likely, we are the kind of people who love to eat cakes, donuts and other goodies. Also likely we are the type of people who do not get regular exercise. Remember the old saying, "use it or lose it"? That saying describes muscles to a tee. Muscles must be used in order to remain big and strong. They also must be fed protein to remain big and strong. Not exercising and not eating enough protein have the same effect on the muscle.

Real people, like us, need lots of complex carbos to meet our energy needs. We also need to make sure we get adequate protein and move our muscles in order to keep them strong. In our opinion, and this is only our opinion, we suggest that you consume about two servings of carbohydrate for every one serving of protein, and plan to get your fat from good food, rather than junk food or added at the table.

Here is Melonie's Food Pyramid. Keep in mind that the carbohydrate level represents complex carbohydrates only.

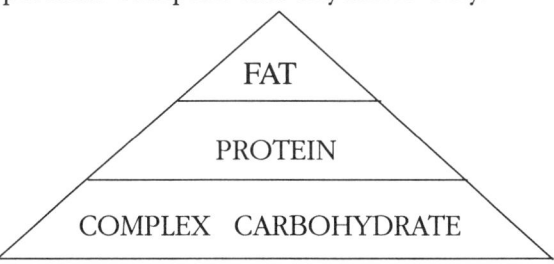

Melonie tries to keep her foodstyle at 25–30 percent protein, 60–65 percent complex carbohydrates and the rest fat. She moves her body a lot. Her muscles need the protein in order to grow bigger and stronger. Remember, too much protein won't hurt you as long as you get enough carbohydrates. To little protein can rob you of precious muscle. In our minds, it's better to err on the side of excess! Not to mention the fact that it makes food planning pretty darn easy! Jan tries to plan her foodstyle at 20 percent protein, 50 percent carbohydrates and 30 percent fat, because she is a BodyLogic freshman! We have consulted several sources that suggest a different proportion: 10 percent protein, 10–30 percent fat, and the remainder complex carbohydrate. You need to pay attention to your body. If you are very out of shape (have little muscle mass) and/or are exercising a lot, you may need a greater quantity than 10 percent protein. You might notice when your protein intake is too low, your muscles don't recover after you have exercised. Leg pain results, and you tend to build muscle mass much more slowly. The goal is not to "bulk up." You don't need to be a body builder.

The more muscle you have, the more fat that is burned when you rest. Muscle uses fat as fuel between meals and when you sleep, as well as during times of stress.

Build your own pyramid

This really is terribly simple once you get the hang of it. Do you remember what it was like learning how to drive a car? Especially if it was a stick shift! Not only did you have to get both feet going in the right order, but you had to do all that stuff with your arms, while looking around watching for other cars (and people), all while remembering every traffic law. Talk about tough! How tough is it now? Hopefully much easier than when you first learned how to drive. Quite likely, driving is done with very little thought, other than trying to avoid an accident. It's the same way building your pyramid and using your pyramid. At first, there are lots of things to think about. Once it becomes habit, all you need to think about is a bit of defensive food planning.

Go back a few chapters and dig up that number you calculated that identifies your caloric need based on activity level. Write that number down: _____

You need to do this calculation only once for now. Later, you can recalculate as your activity level or body weight change. Here we go with the math again. We'll show you an example or two first, then you can build your own pyramid.

Example: For the sake of simplicity, let's say you calculated a basic caloric need of 3,000 calories per day, and you decided to go whole-hog and try to keep your calories at 10 percent fat.

1) Fat

Total calories = 3000 x 10% (fat% you want) = 300 fat calories. Knowing each gram of fat contains 9 calories, we simply divide 300 by 9 to get about 33 fat grams.

2) Protein

Total calories = 3,000 minus 300 (fat calories) = 2,700. (Hey, leftovers!)

Leftovers = 2700 x 30% (% of protein) = 810 protein calories. Knowing there are 4 calories to each gram of protein, divide 810 by 4 = about 202 protein grams.

You can choose to count protein grams or live by numbers of servings instead. (You can also choose how much protein you want in your diet, but never go below 10 percent, preferably not below 15–20 percent.) It just depends on how much structure you need. In the beginning, you may need more structure than later. If you choose to live life without obsession, one serving of protein is 12–16 grams. Let's use 16. Divide 202 by 16 = 12 servings of protein per day. For example, two ounces of water-pack tuna provides 16 grams of protein! Who eats just two ounces of anything? Average serving sizes of meats are three or four ounces. If you eat four ounces, that constitutes two of your protein servings for the day!

This does not mean that you should eat twelve servings of meat a day. Many foods are mixed, they have both protein and carbohydrate. For example, every two slices of whole wheat bread provides 4 grams of protein, or one-fourth of a serving. Same thing with a couple of ears of corn. Dried beans, peas and nuts also contain large amounts of protein. Most dairy products are good sources of protein. Don't become stressed, we gave you a chart as to what constitutes a serving for many different foods, most of which don't come with food labels. (Look in the back of the book.)

3) Carbohydrates: This is the easiest calculation. It's the leftover leftovers.

Leftover calories = 2,700 minus 810 (protein calories) = 1,890 carbohydrate calories. Again there are 4 calories per gram of carbo. So divide 1,890 by 4 = 472 carbohydrate grams. Think again of 12–16 grams of carbohydrate per serving. We will use 16. So, 472 divided by 16 = 29 carbohydrate servings. For example, one quarter cup of uncooked eight-grain hot cereal provides 20 grams of carbo. That's a little more than one serving. Two slices of whole wheat bread provides 25 grams—that's almost two servings. Half of a large banana provides about 15 grams, that's about one serving. Rounding out the numbers, this typical breakfast, not including milk, would give you about four carbohydrate servings. Have a cup of milk and you probably have about five. Then you will have three snacks and two more meals during the day. It's easy to get those twenty-nine servings.

That's the beauty of this system. If you work with servings, you do it to make sure you are getting your minimum needs met. You may be quite happy just eating complex carbos if you don't enjoy meat that much. If this is the case you will have to force yourself to get your protein from the right sources. A person can only eat so many servings of rice and beans in order to get complete protein out of the deal. This is our system. We make sure we get at least one serving of high protein food each meal, whether it be dairy or very lean meat. If we don't make it, we supplement the daily intake with a milk shake made with vanilla flavor protein powder, the kind without fat or sugar. If you are still hungry, anything extra you eat is icing on the cake. (Don't take that literally, unless it's Mel's icing recipe!) In a short amount of time, you will be able to recognize what a balanced meal looks like, and what your best sources of low-fat protein are. Remember that some vegetables and all beans and legumes contain quite a bit of carbo and protein. Double the bang for the buck.

Again, it's all about balance. Get your carbs from a variety of fruits, veggies, whole grains, beans, legumes, and low-fat or nonfat dairy. Try to eat four to five veggies and two to three fresh fruits per day, and at least two servings of dairy per day. Limit the carbs from sweets, white flour, white rice, pasta made with white flour and starchy veggies like potatoes and corn. Try whole wheat pasta or spelt grain pasta. They really taste great and satisfy you much more. Try to eat brown and wild rice instead of white, and the longer it takes to cook, the better it is. Shorter cooking times on rice and beans means convenience, but it also means that a lot of the nutritional value and fiber have been processed out.

Get your protein from nonfat dairy and lean cuts of meat, or from dried peas, beans and legumes. Limit protein from higher fat sources like regular cheese, peanut butter, and typical junk foods. Eat this way and you will hardly need to watch the fat grams. Keep your food plate filled with one third protein and two-thirds complex carbo. Easy? Yup! Still hungry? Great! You are doing it right! High-octane fuel takes more energy to digest and use than foods that have already been processed once. In other words, you burn more calories when you eat better quality fuel. The more high-octane gas in your tank, the more energy the body expends to use that energy, and the more energy your body needs to keep burning all of that high-octane fuel.

If you are still hungry after a meal, add more complex carbos, starting with fruits and whole grains, dried peas, beans, legumes, even brown or wild rice. Reserve more refined products like breads as the last thing you eat to try to fill up on. When hunger strikes, and you have met all of your basic needs, you can eat some fat-free or ultra low-fat protein, such as fat-free turkey slices or water-pack tuna, or even boiled shrimp. Be cautious though. Processed meats and fish tend to contain a lot of salt. Salt means fluid retention and bloating.

Even splurge on some of Mel's Fudge Brownies (see recipe in the "Pleasurable Side Trips" chapter) if you know you have met all of your needs for the day. Think of breads, cakes, cookies and other floury things as dessert. Remember what your mother always told you? "When you clean your plate (or at least eat your veggies) you can have dessert." If your mom didn't say that, we would bet your grandmother did!

OK. How about another example with a bit less narration! Estimated caloric need is 2,200 calories per day, at 10 percent calories from fat. That's Mel! You can relate.

1. Fat: 2,200 x 10% = 220 fat calories divided by 9 = 24 grams of fat. Fat is about 12 grams per serving. We're not sure who established that one. At any rate, it's more labor intensive to count fat by servings, because there are such varying amounts in most everything we eat. Not to mention those labels that say "0" grams of fat, yet list "canola oil" on the label? Doesn't make sense? It does because the government does not require the label to list anything less than one fat gram. So, a food serving could contain .99 grams of fat. If the food contains 50 calories, that's almost 18 percent of calories from fat. Not fair, is it? Become a label-reading maniac.

2. Protein: 2,200 - 220 = 1,980. (Hey, leftovers again.) 1980 x 30% = 594, divided by 4 = 148 protein grams. 148 divided by 16 = about 9 servings of protein for the day.

3. Carbohydrate: 1,980 (leftovers!) - 594 = 1,386 (leftover, leftovers!). 1,386 divided by 4 = 346 carbohydrate grams. 346 divided by 16 = about 22 carbo servings.

Now you calculate your own pyramid:

1. Fat: _____ Start with your basic caloric need. You just wrote it down a few pages ago.

x _____% Your desired percentage of calories from fat.

divide by 9 =_____ Number of grams of fat for the day.

2. Protein: _____Leftovers! Total calories minus fat calories.

x   30% = _____ Number of protein calories.

divide by 4 = _____ **Number of protein grams.**

divide by 16 = _____ Number of protein servings per day minimum!

3. Carbohydrate: _____ Leftover leftovers! Total leftovers minus protein calories = carbohydrate calories.

divide by 4 = _____ **Number of carbohydrate grams.**

divide by 16 = _____ Number of carbohydrate servings per day minimum!

This is your road map. You will find detours on a daily basis. It is up to you to decide how to structure your meals to get all of your needs met. If you don't like lower-fat, high-protein foods for breakfast, eat whole-grain cereals, fruit, maybe even nonfat yogurt for breakfast. Eat some whole-grain pancakes or whole wheat French toast made with egg substitute. (If you don't like egg substitute, use egg whites.) If breakfast is less than your desired percentage of protein, try to make it up during the rest of the day. If today you are craving carbos and go a bit overboard, do the opposite and hit the protein a bit heavier the next day. There are no hard and fast rules. You can be as structured or unstructured as you want, just make sure your needs are met. Here's the challenge, need some protein but crave sweet carbos? Eat one of Mel's Fudge Brownies! They are well balanced, with 13 grams of carbo, 6 grams of protein, essentially no fat and no sugar! (Make them with whole wheat flour for added nutrition.) See, you can have your cake and eat your protein, too!

We keep it all straight this way. Our bodies need at least one good serving of protein at breakfast or we are starving all day and have difficulty getting enough protein the rest of the day. We also take our activity breaks in the morning, right after breakfast. Our breakfasts contain something from each food group, something from each level of Mel's pyramid, and average 400–600 calories. They contain 1–2 protein servings, and the balance of the calories comes from complex carbos.

Here's an example of a balanced breakfast: Two nonfat egg-substitute scrambled eggs, cooked with one ounce of low-fat or nonfat cheese or turkey ham and butter flavor spray. Also, one and one-half whole-wheat English muffins with nonfat, fruit-flavored cream cheese on two, and one and one-half teaspoons of reduced-fat peanut butter on one (if you opted for the nonfat cheese in the eggs). If you got the fat with the cheese or the turkey ham, then it's more nonfat cream cheese or fruit spread for muffin half number three. Also have a good serving of fresh fruit in season. You can vary this breakfast when you are really lazy and have half a cup or so of low-fat or nonfat cottage cheese instead of the eggs, maybe even put the fruit on top of the cottage cheese! That's not so difficult is it? You will find many sample menus in a later chapter. We just wanted to ease your mind. Do the math once and you don't have to do it again until you decide it's time to change your caloric intake level. This is a very easy way to plan your foodstyle. After a few years, you will reach for breakfasts like these without any more thought than you reach for the croissants, Danish or doughnuts today.

Ever tried a Monte Cristo sandwich? Make it with nonfat turkey and nonfat or low-fat cheese! Wonderful for breakfast! It is simply a French toast "sandwich" stuffed with a low-fat ham or turkey and low-fat or nonfat cheese just prior to grilling. How about an egg and cheese muffin? The point is this: Breakfast can be made fast and nutritious. It's probably the easiest and definitely the most important meal of the day. Make up a large batch of whole-grain hot cereal when you have the time, stick it in the fridge, and microwave it for breakfasts or snacks during the week when you don't have time to cook. Try the good old-fashioned, slow-cooking oatmeal, or better yet, steel-cut oats. So much more flavor, and talk about satisfying! Brown rice is a grain. Got some leftovers? Microwave them and stir in some cinnamon, sweetener and unsweetened applesauce. Yummy!

In five minutes you can whip up an egg and cheese muffin, grab a piece of fruit and you have breakfast on the run. You can make up pancakes ahead, keep them in the fridge, and either "nuke" them in the microwave or put them in the toaster. Spread with fruit spread or applesauce and presto, another breakfast on the run. Works with waffles and French toast, too! It just takes a little practice and a bit of creativity!

Now all you have to do is decide how you want to spread your pyramid out through your day's three meals and three snacks. That doesn't mean you can't have four or six snacks. Start with three. If you are needing to eat more than every two and one-half to three hours, then you should be increasing your meal size just a bit and make sure you are getting enough complex carbos, fat and protein in those meals! If you are not needing snacks, then you are either eating too many calories at meal time, or you are consuming too much fat and not enough complex carbo. If you are eating high-octane fuel and in the right proportions, you should be needing to eat every three hours or so. Your body needs at least a serving of complex carbos between meals to keep that metabolic flame burning!

Three weeks into her lifestyle change, Jan complained that she was waking up hungry during the night. She gets an A+++! That means she is eating the right balance of foods. The only thing she needs to do is make sure she gets her bedtime snack and her problem will be solved.

If we have not yet convinced you to eat breakfast before you leave the house, and to pack a sack lunch whenever possible, check out the next chapter on fast food! You will be amazed at what some of those "healthier" fast-food options really contain!

Give this way of eating the good old college try. What have you got to lose except fat, fatigue and illness? More importantly, you will gain muscle, strength, energy and improve your overall health.

Here's one more final word of wisdom, likely one of the most important things we will ever tell you. Good food may cost more in some instances, but your body will run better and longer on it. It's cheaper than health insurance deductibles and losing your ability to work due to poor health. Spending a bit more for good quality food will save you money in the long run. Just keep in mind that most quality foods are in their natural state, and less expensive than their processed counterparts. So you see, you save money either way when you eat good food! You might then respond by saying, "What about the time to fix more natural foods?" It takes no longer to whip up a bowl of ten-minute eight-grain cereal than it does to brew a pot of coffee, and you can do both while washing your face in the morning. It takes no longer to fix your own version of fast food than it does to sit in line at the drive-through during lunch hour. What good is extra time if you are too sick to enjoy it, or worse yet, dead? Have we made our point?

Balance your meals. Give your body what it needs. Consume high octane fuel and love every bite of it. That's BodyLogic!

Your positive self statement for today: I am what I eat. I am whole and complete!

Life in the Fast Lane

The Fat Facts About Fast Food

We promised you in one of the early chapters that eating out does not have to be an unhealthy or irritating experience. We all find ourselves on the road, starving to death and having forgot to put munchies in the car, for whatever reason. If you have ever been to Portland or Seattle, you know what our traffic jams are like. Plan an hour to get somewhere and you will need one and one-half to two hours. So much for lunch! And your body needs fuel! What to do?

The easiest thing if you have ten minutes to spare is to pop into a grocery store that has a salad bar and/or a deli. Create your own salad and top with the low-fat or fat-free dressing. Skip the cheese and ham. Toss on some turkey. Pick through the hard-cooked eggs and get just the egg white. Toss on some beans and lots of veggies. Then go to the bakery and grab a sourdough or whole-wheat roll, even a whole grain bagel. Instead of bread, go over to the deli and order a turkey sandwich on whole wheat bread with mustard, lettuce and tomato, no mayo or cheese. Then pop over to produce and grab a banana or other piece of fruit and you have a decent lunch on the run. Grab some nonfat granola bars or pretzels to keep in the car.

So you have all of ten minutes to grab a bite, find a place to park and get to your appointment on time? All that's around is a "fat" food place? Here's what you will face. Even the so-called healthier items can be loaded with fat. Do the best you can and plan to watch the fat grams for the rest of the day, as well as the next day. You can do fairly well if you research in advance. When you do have time and are out and about, pop into several of the major chain places and ask for a brochure outlining the nutritional information of the various menu items. Pull out your highlighter and mark those selections that fit your body's needs. Stick it behind the sun visor or in the glove box of your car, and you will always be prepared. You can also pop into a local bookstore. There are several books that list only nutritional counts of various fast foods. But if you are like us, and need to clean out the glove box or failed to plan ahead, here are some typical fast-food items and their nutritional information. Keep in mind the numbers vary somewhat from restaurant to restaurant. In most cases, you can ask to have dressings left off of salads and sandwiches, and hold the sour cream on a baked potato. See if they have a low-fat, or fat-free ranch dressing instead. That works great on dry sandwiches and plain, baked potatoes!

Note: The following are provided as examples only. Nutritional information is obtained from the United States Department of Agriculture (USDA), and we have used the averages of many different restaurants. Nutritional content may vary for many reasons. Please check with your local restaurants for the most up-to-date nutritional information on their menu selections.

Ice cream/frozen goodies

Vanilla Soft-Serve Ice Cream or "Fake" Ice Cream (½ cup):

Calories:	174	
Protein:	3	
Carb:	20	
Fat:	**9**	**(48%)**

Frozen Yogurt, Non-Fat (½ cup):

Calories:	102	
Protein:	5	
Carb:	20	
Fat:	**0**	**(0%)**

Mel has been known, on a very hot day, to order up a large serving of frozen yogurt for lunch. I know, no fruits or veggies, hardly food in its natural state, but in a pinch, it is fairly well-balanced and you can't beat the fat grams. It will satisfy you for a couple of hours or so. Sometimes that's all it takes to get you through that one meeting until you can get some real food. For those of you who are lactose intolerant, we have discovered something quite amazing. Yogurt that comes from the chain restaurants and stores does not cause us the upset that the frozen yogurt bought in a grocery store does. Makes you wonder if some frozen yogurt has any real dairy in it.

Sandwiches

Grilled Chicken Sandwich (one sandwich):

Calories: 426

Protein: 27

Carb: 38

Fat: **19**   **(40%)**

Ask them to hold the mayo or dressing and you will drop that fat down into a tolerable range by Mel's standards. Skip the fries and order a garden salad (no cheese or pick off the cheese) with low-cal dressing on the side.

Fried Chicken Sandwich (one sandwich):

Calories: 515

Protein: 24

Carb: 39

Fat: **30**   **(52.9%)** We would rather starve!

Typical Roast Beef Sandwich (one sandwich):

Calories: 446

Protein: 26

Carb: 34

Fat: **19**   **(48%)** You can do better. These numbers are for a plain, regular-size sandwich, no cheese!

Veggie Pocket Sandwich (one sandwich):

Calories: 306

Protein: 9

Carb: 45

Fat: **10**   **(30%)** It's the cheese and the dressing that destroys it! The chicken version adds more fat.

Regular Hamburger (one sandwich):

Calories: 248

Protein: 13

Carb: 21

Fat: **12**   **(44%)** Without cheese!

Double-meat, double-cheese burger (one sandwich):

Calories:	600	
Protein:	31	
Carb:	41	
Fat:	**35**	**(53%)**

Quarter-pound burger with cheese (one sandwich):

Calories:	630	
Protein:	28	
Carb:	39	
Fat:	**38**	**(54%)**

Small, deli-style turkey sub, no cheese (one sandwich):

Calories:	218	
Protein:	12	
Carb:	34	
Fat:	**4**	**(16%)** We'd say go for it! Hold the mayo and substitute mustard!

Regular turkey sandwich on wheat bread, sub-style, (one sandwich):

Calories:	288	
Protein:	17	
Carb:	45	
Fat:	**4**	**(12.5%)** Even Mel would eat that one in a heartbeat!

Pizza

If you are lucky, you can find a place that does personal-size pizzas. Ask for a veggie with no cheese, then put a sprinkle of Parmesan on the top. You'll really save on the fat.

Veggie—12-inch thin crust pizza, serving = about ⅓ pizza

Calories:	320	
Protein:	14	
Carb:	37	
Fat:	**13**	**(37%)**

Salads

Typical pasta salad (one serving):

Calories:	243	
Protein:	6	
Carb:	21	
Fat:	**15**	**(56%)**

Broiled chicken salad (one salad):

Calories:	200	
Protein:	23	
Carb:	8	
Fat:	**9**	**(40%)** And that does not include the breadstick! Ask for nonfat dressing and hold the cheese, and you will do much better.

Garden salad (one salad):

Calories:	97	
Protein:	6	
Carb:	8	
Fat:	**5**	**(46%)** That darn cheese again!

French fries (one regular-size) order:

Calories:	400	
Protein:	5	
Carb:	36	
Fat:	**20**	**(45%)**

Imagine how much fat you swallow with a typical fried-chicken sandwich and an order of fries! And watch serving sizes. A "regular" order of fries at one store has almost the same nutritional counts as a "medium" order at another.)

Quick Breads/Muffins

Low-fat muffin (one muffin):

Calories:	205	
Protein:	3	
Carbo:	44	
Fat:	**3**	**(13%)**
Sugars:	33	Other than the sugar, way to go!

Powdered cake-doughnut (one doughnut)

Calories:	191	
Protein:	3	
Carb:	23	
Fat:	**10**	**(47%)**
Sugars:	12	

Look at the doughnut versus the muffin. The muffin's carbohydrates come almost entirely from sugar as compared to the doughnut. Isn't that amazing? Not really. We warned you about ready-made low-fat goodies. Watch that sugar content. Your pancreas will not like it one bit.

Tacos

Chicken, soft taco (one taco):

Calories:	185	
Protein:	8	
Carb:	21	
Fat:	**8**	**(39%)** Overall, not so bad. Not much chicken in there though!

Regular soft taco with beef (one taco):

Calories:	205	
Protein:	10	
Carb:	17	
Fat:	**11**	**(48%)**

Breakfasts

Breakfast biscuit, plain (one sandwich):

Calories:	295	
Protein:	18	
Carb:	28	
Fat:	**13**	**(40%)**

Bacon, egg and cheese biscuit (one sandwich):

Calories:	580	
Protein:	26	
Carb:	42	
Fat:	**34**	**(53%)**

Sausage biscuit (one sandwich):
Calories: 595
Protein: 19
Carb: 43
Fat: **39**   **(59%)**

Pancakes, plain (one serving):
Calories: 295
Protein: 9
Carb: 54
Fat: **5**   **(15%)** Not bad! This does not in-
                                   clude butter or syrup, just the pan-
                                   cakes dry!

French toast sticks, 1 serving:
Calories: 465
Protein: 7
Carb: 56
Fat: **24**   **(46%)** Make Mel's version instead!
                                   (See recipe on page 188.) It won't
                                   take any longer than waiting in line
                                   at the drive-thru!

Chicken
Regular fried-chicken breast with skin (one-half breast):
Calories: 303
Protein: 22
Carb: 12
Fat: **18**   **(53%)**

Chicken bites (one order, about six pieces with BBQ sauce):
Calories: 330
Protein: 17
Carb: 25
Fat: **18**   **(49%)** Pretty amazing, huh?

Regular-style roasted, one-half chicken breast with skin:
Calories: 193
Protein: 29
Carb: 0
Fat: **8**   **(37%)**

This list is far from exhaustive. It is yet another tool to help you with making small but significant changes in the way you eat. A little detective work yields some huge payoffs! We were surprised by some of the numbers. Were you? You can eat out, and you can eat fast food. Just use your head and plan ahead. That's BodyLogic!

Backfires

The Tootn' Scooties!

Birds do it, bees do it, even you and me just sometimes gotta do it!

Beans, beans, the musical fruit
The more we eat, the more we toot—
The more we toot, the more they avoid us
So misunderstood, the source of that flatus!

Gas, gas, quiet or loud
Who was the source of that little green cloud?
They hum, they run, they fan, they look away
To relieve it in public is a disgrace, they say!

So little studied, this natural thing
Eat good food and it will sing!
Don't pop a pill, it will rescind
Just eat slow and stop sucking wind!

(Neither one of us will admit to writing this one, but one of us did!)

Have we given you enough clues about the topic of this chapter? So many people complain about this problem, yet it remains one of the most socially unacceptable things out there! To be honest with you, we think a productive cough or blowing one's nose in public is much more disgusting. At least a little gas event doesn't splash germy bodily fluids on one's neighbor! Sure, it may be momentarily unpleasant, but no real harm is done, is there? Besides, passing a bit of gas at the right moment might just be self-defense in some situations! Mother Nature gave skunks that quality, did she perhaps do something similar with human beings? The poor skunk is always getting a bad rap, too.

One thing we did not mention in the food chapters is the fact that your body may respond to your new foodstyle, shall we say, with a bang! If you eat high-quality foods, expect to experience some extra gas production, not to mention some irregularity. For most people, this will resolve, as your body adapts to its new fuel source. Trust us, it also works in reverse. After you have been giving your body quality fuel for a long time, and then you consume one high-fat meal, guess what happens? The Tootn' Scooties all over again! This is simply the result of the body's response to having to digest substances it is not accustomed to digesting.

Call it what you will, but the medical terms for this malady are flatus and flatulence. Such polite terms, aren't they?

So, what if you have gas, but you haven't changed your foodstyle for a long time? There actually has been quite a lot of medical research done on the subject. Complaints of excess gas are the number one reasons people see gastroenterologists each year. In most cases, gas is not a symptom of a serious problem, and seldom causes damage to anyone other than to some people who attempt to ignite the stuff. Yes, it can actually be flammable! Please don't try this. Why disfigure that beautiful bottom of yours?

Of course, the social consequences are less than desirable. Did you know that in some ancient cultures, it was illegal to pass gas in public? Did you know that Hippocrates investigated gas production extensively? Even Ben Franklin struggled with finding the cure for tootn'! In Franklin's proposal to the Royal Academy in Brussels, 1770, he wrote: "Were it not for the obviously offensive smell accompanying such escapes, polite people would probably be under no more restraint in discharging such wind in company than they are in spitting or blowing their noses.

"My question therefore should be: To discover some drug, wholesome and not disagreeable, to be mixed with our common food or sauces, that shall render the natural discharges of wind from our bodies not only inoffensive, but agreeable as perfumes."

The Guinness World Book of Records keeps track of the greatest number of times any one person has passed wind within a twenty-four-hour period! (Hey, *Guinness*, get a life!)

Interestingly though, passing gas through belching is actually considered a compliment to the cook in some cultures. In King Henry

VIII's time, a loud burp was commonplace. In the Middle Eastern culture of today a burp is considered a gesture of appreciation for a meal. However, we were unable to find any culture that socially accepts passing wind from the back door. So why is such a natural thing such a social stigma in our society today? Probably for the same reason picking one's nose is. If the majority of people consider it to be unacceptable, then it must be unacceptable. Guess you could call that PeopleLogic.

Like the wind, you can't see it, but you certainly know it is there.

Research studies have found that the average person generates anywhere from one to eight cups of gas every day. This gas must be passed in some way. Unfortunately, these events often occur at the worst possible time, in the worst possible place and when least expected. For many of us, these events are not within our control. Researchers have found that the average person has anywhere from ten to thirty passing events per day! There are some very real physiological causes for gas. There are emotional causes as well.

The source can be determined by the location of the noise. Think of your mouth as the "muffler" (because you can control the volume of noise that comes out of it). Think of your bottom as the "amplifier." Belching comes from the muffler: It is produced from swallowed air. Gas passing through the back door comes from the amplifier.

Belching can be easily reduced by watching what things you put in your mouth and the rate at which those substances get to the stomach. Try not to eat too quickly. Scarfing down a meal means you swallow a lot of air with that meal. Eating more slowly will reduce the amount of air that is trapped with your food. Carbonated beverages contain carbon dioxide—GAS. Limit the number of carbonated beverages you consume, and when you do consume them, drink slowly. Chewing gum and smoking, not to mention wearing dentures that do not fit properly also can result in swallowed air. If you are prone to belching, avoid chewing gum and smoking. If you wear dentures, see your dentist or denturist to make sure they are fitting properly. Other sources of air swallowing can be postnasal drip, a dry mouth, or any activity with the mouth that results in frequent swallowing. Some people swallow air when they are nervous.

Have you ever been on a plane and found your ears to be plugged? What are the things that relieve the plugged feeling? Chewing gum, swallowing or yawning, all of which produce swallowed air. For those of you who tend to be gassy after an airplane trip, it may not have been caused by all of that wonderful food you ate on board. Fortunately, relieving gas through belching is fairly socially acceptable. If you find your belching to be excessive, bothersome or associated with a feeling of bloating or abdominal pain, you should see your doctor. Your problem may be due to stress or lifestyle, but in rare instances it can be an indication of a more serious problem. Over the counter medications may be OK for occasional problems (check with your doctor first), but long term use of these medications may mask a true health problem.

So what about "back-door" events? Back-door gas usually comes from the colon, and is caused by the digestion of food. Simple carbohydrates (like sugar, potatoes, white flour and white rice) may not be completely digested in the small intestine. Another simple sugar which is often a culprit is milk sugar, or lactose. A fair percentage of people do not have the enzyme lactase which is required to break down milk sugar. These people have a condition called lactose intolerance. Both of your authors are lactose intolerant. When foods containing simple carbos reach the colon, undigested sugars are fermented by the bacteria that normally live there. This fermentation may result in gas, much like the fermentation of fruit results in a bottle of bubbly.

We all have heard that beans will cause back-door gas. Let's give credit where credit is due. Beans are your friend. They are high in fiber and protein. It's not the poor bean's fault that you end up tootn'! Blame it on your body. According to researchers, beans contain a special kind of sugar which is a complex rather than simple carbohydrate. These sugars cannot be absorbed by the human body. The human body does not have the enzymes necessary to fully digest these substances. So you see, it really is the fault of your own body, not the beans. Fortunately, there are products on the market that will give you what nature forgot. Beano is a popular product that provides the enzymes necessary to help break down the sugars found in beans and other legumes. Taken with the first bite of the offending food, Beano or a similar product will often reduce or eliminate the unpleasantries you would otherwise expect. You no longer have to plan bean meals when you know you will not be in public for a day or two. Eat your beans and be social. Eat your beans and watch that fat burn!

Besides beans, milk and simple carbos, many people experience difficulty after consuming fruits and vegetables. No one should eliminate fruits and veggies just because they cause gas. If onions give you problems, and beans give you problems, try some Beano before you eat that chili. Beano works on beans, as well as veggies. If you have problems with dairy foods, try taking some lactase enzyme tablets with the first bite of dairy. You can find them in natural food stores, or they are sold in grocery and drug stores under the name Lactaid. There are also dairy products on the market that have lactase enzyme added to them. Look for them. You might pay a bit more but they are less expensive than buying all of those pills.

These tips will help you reduce or eliminate unpleasant emissions:

1. Avoid soda pop and other carbonated beverages.
2. Limit gum chewing and sucking on hard candy.
3. Avoid smoking and chewing tobacco.
4. Try to reduce your stress level.
5. Eat slowly and don't talk with your mouth full! Didn't your mother always tell you that? She knew what she was talking about!
6. Get plenty of exercise. Physical activity speeds up the digestive process and aids in more rapid elimination of excess gas.
7. Take a walk after your meal. It has the same effect as burping a baby after it is fed. If you enjoy this only in your own company, you can let your muffler and amplifier do their jobs without embarrassment.
8. Reduce your dairy intake or better yet, start taking lactase enzyme tablets. Nonfat dairy is an excellent source of protein. You don't want to eliminate dairy if you can control the problem some other way (or unless you are allergic to it).
9. Avoid sorbitol and fructose, sugars often found in carbonated beverages, candies and many other processed foods.
10. Continue to eat foods high in fiber, but try using canned/cooked fruits and veggies for a while. Cooking helps to break down some of those carbos before they hit the colon. For some unknown reason, many people find fewer problems with gas if they eat beans, veggies and other high fiber foods on a regular basis. Kind of blows hot air at the theory of the researchers, doesn't it?

11. Be on the lookout for soybeans and soybean products. These can be some of the worst offenders. Plan ahead, and have Beano on hand!

12. Try to avoid extensive use of antibiotics if at all possible. Antibiotics may kill some of the gas-producing bacteria, but they also kill the good bacteria as well. Upsetting the natural balance of the colon can have some serious side effects. Let nature take its course when you get a minor cold. Remember, most colds and flu are caused by viruses. Antibiotics only kill bacteria. They do nothing to viruses! So the next time you get a cold or flu, put your money into a good bowl of chicken soup and crank up the heat on the electric blanket! Skip the trip to the doctor to beg for antibiotics unless you are clearly getting worse rather than better after two to three days.

13. Many over-the-counter preparations are available to help ease the symptoms of gas, but many can cause constipation and other gastrointestinal difficulties. Often times the more natural remedies are the most soothing. Most people find peppermint tea, or very strong peppermint candies (like Altoids) to be helpful. Activated charcoal capsules can be found in health food stores. They absorb the gas like a sponge!

14. The best treatment is prevention. Try lactase enzyme with the first bite of dairy. Take Beano with the first bite of beans or veggies that are known to give you problems.

Finally, if your problems are not relieved by these self-help measures, and you have abdominal pain and/or chronic diarrhea or constipation, or are under a doctor's care for any reason, see your doctor.

The next time you start Tootn' don't blame all of that high-octane food. It is not necessarily the high-octane gas causing all of *your* gas!

Beans, beans that musical fruit,
The more you eat the less you toot!
The less you toot, the less you blush.
Eat more beans, your body will adjust!
(Neither of us will fess up to writing that
variation-on-a-theme either!)

**Your positive self statement for today: My body is
my shrine. I love the way it looks, I love the way it
feels, and I love the way it sounds!**

The Rules of the Road

Helpful Hints

For fat-free baking, substitute an equal amount of fat-free sour cream, mayonnaise, or unsweetened applesauce for the fat. You may need to adjust the liquids down a bit. In recipes calling for any type of liquid, use powdered buttermilk (1 fat gram per three tablespoons) mixed with one cup of water and replace the liquid measure for measure. *The most important lesson in cooking: In order to reduce or eliminate fat, you must replace it with moisture and texture and taste!*

In recipes like some baked goods that are a batter or dough before baking or cooking, try substituting some low-fat cottage cheese, blended to "de-curd" it. Use an equal measure of low-fat cottage cheese to replace the combined measure of eggs and oil or fat.

You may need to reduce the other liquid a bit. Experiment!

If you want to reduce or eliminate sugar in baking, substitute one and one-fourth measures of unsweetened applesauce for each measure of sugar. Adjust the liquids down a bit if necessary to compensate for the added moisture of the applesauce. If you like a sweeter taste, six packets or teaspoons of NutraSweet equals one-fourth cup of sugar. Add Barley Malt or fruit-based liquid sweetener measure for measure for the sugar, though fruit-based sweetener is a bit more detectable than the Barley Malt. Barley Malt has a mild flavor that reminds us of molasses. Use fresh fruits, fruit spread, applesauce or fruit yogurt to top pancakes, waffles or French toast. We think this is much more nutritious and satisfying than artificially sweetened syrups. Top hot or cold cereal with fresh fruit or applesauce instead of sugar. Fruit yogurt also goes well with some cold cereals, especially low-fat granolas and Grape Nuts.

Instead of using oil to grease baking pans or cookware, use a bit of spray oil. You can sauté in a bit of low-sodium, fat-free chicken, beef or vegetable broth.

If you like rice, but are short on time, make it up on the weekend and keep it in the fridge to reheat as needed or add to casseroles during the week! Reheated brown rice (especially short grain) makes a wonderful, nutty hot cereal when topped with some unsweetened applesauce, cinnamon and a bit of NutraSweet. Nothing will satisfy you more or keep you going longer than brown rice. Brown rice has more flavor, more fiber and more nutrition than regular white rice. You will feel twice as full after eating brown rice, and it will stay with you longer. Try it a few times and you'll be hooked!

To cook skinless, boneless chicken breasts, turkey loins, low-fat varieties of fish, or extra-lean cuts of beef or pork: Season as desired with herbs, buffalo-wing powder seasoning, any type of powdered seasoning that has less than 1 gram of fat per serving. Do whatever you like. Place the meat in a baking bag, close it up, and place in a baking dish so the meat is all in one layer. Bake at 350 degrees for thirty minutes (for chicken or turkey breast), using the second rack spot up from the bottom of the oven. The meat comes out very tender and juicy, so tender you can cut it with a fork. Isn't that amazing? Experiment with different meats and different quantities of meat. Remember, keep the moisture and the flavor, lose the fat! Mel uses baking bags to prepare most of her meats.

You can try mixing powdered butter substitute with water to get butter flavor into your recipes, however, we have not had much success with this approach. Try pouring in some nonfat liquid butter spray. Experiment with butter-flavored extract, nut or vanilla or coffee extracts, or lemon or orange zest in your baked goods instead.

Thicken sauces, soups and gravies with a mixture of cornstarch or arrowroot and water. When making fruit pies or cobblers, put some uncooked tapioca or flavored or unflavored, unsweetened gelatin with the fruit to thicken the juices.

Instead of traditional pie crust, try egg roll or wonton wrappers layered, or even some phyllo dough, or try a mixture of Grape Nuts cereal with just a bit of Barley Malt to hold it together. You can also create a nice crumb topping using a mixture of uncooked oatmeal and Barley Malt. When the dessert has cooled half way or so, sprinkle on some Grape Nuts cereal or steel-cut oats on top of the crumb topping to add that nutty taste and texture.

Use nonfat evaporated milk in recipes that call for a traditional white sauce. Thicken with a mixture of corn starch and water. If the cream sauce is cheese based, nonfat or low-fat cheese will also provide some thickening.

In baked goods calling for melted chocolate, substitute cocoa powder mixed with water. You will need to experiment with the amount of flour to compensate for loss in thickness of the chocolate.

Toss fruit salads with fruit yogurt or a combination of nonfat mayonnaise and sugar substitute and perhaps some lemon or orange zest, or use a splash of lemon, orange or pineapple juice.

Fat-free cream cheese does not hold up as well as its fat-laden counterparts in baked goods or in chilled dessert recipes. The exception is Mel's icing, because she uses some special tricks to make it perfect! Instead, put some nonfat or low-fat ricotta in a blender with a bit of plain yogurt or nonfat mayonnaise and blend it until smooth. Low-fat or nonfat cottage cheese blended until creamy is also a good substitute for cream cheese in recipes.

To make glazes for vegetables or meats, thicken with a bit of tapioca, cornstarch or arrowroot mixed with water.

Use one-fourth cup of egg substitute wherever one egg is called for. You can substitute egg whites as well. If you like scrambled eggs, but hate scrambled egg substitute, throw in a teaspoon or so of nonfat butter-flavor spray (in the refrigerator section of your grocery store). You will taste good old-fashioned buttery flavored scrambled eggs, you will get a lot of protein, and you won't miss the fat. To add even more flavor, melt some nonfat cheese over the top or throw it in while the eggs are cooking. Toss in some cooked turkey ham or sauteed vegetables to give it flavor.

Cut the fat content in half in meat recipes by using one-half the amount of ground meat and substitute the other half with brown rice or a crumbled meat substitute.

When making soups like bean or split pea, use turkey ham instead of regular ham. Cut the total amount of meat in half and add some Liquid Smoke to taste. Not only do you save fat grams, but you also save money.

Use imitation bacon bits or wherever real bacon is called for. If you like real bacon, substitute turkey bacon!

In meat loaf or other meat recipes that call for eggs to provide moisture, add a cup or so of finely chopped mushrooms. You won't find a moister meat loaf anywhere! You can also use an egg substitute.

Get some protein into that stir-fry veggie recipe with some chopped low-fat tofu. Trust us, you won't notice any change in the flavor at all. The tofu takes on the flavor of whatever it's with. It gives an extra protein boost to the meal without all of the fat of meat.

You can experiment by using low-fat tofu in recipes in place of cream cheese.

Substitute carob chips for chocolate chips in baked goodies.

Instead of putting traditional icing on cake or brownies, top just before serving with fat-free, sugar-free pudding and some fat-free whipped topping. This tastes so rich and creamy!

To make "fried chicken," dip a skinless boneless chicken "boob" in some egg substitute, then into some seasoned bread crumbs or crushed corn flakes, or fat-free herb blend Parmesan cheese, or corn meal, or flour followed by a second dipping in the egg (or whatever you like!). Place the chicken in a baking dish lightly spray oiled. Bake at 350–375 degrees for thirty to forty-five minutes or until done.

To make "french fries," slice up fresh potatoes (or use frozen ones) and place them on a lightly spray-oiled or nonstick baking sheet. Season with salt, barbecue or Cajun spices, ranch, onion or garlic salad dressing mix, fat-free Parmesan, or whatever you like. Bake at 400 degrees until golden. Turn and bake the other side to brown if necessary.

If you like peanut butter, try mixing one half your usual amount with an equal part of nonfat cream cheese. You will retain all the flavor and texture, but lose half the fat.

Get creative. Have fun. Often the first attempt at a substitution will not give the result you want. Just feed it to the cat (OK, we're prejudiced!) and keep trying! You might just luck out and stumble upon something truly incredible. Most of all, love your food and enjoy every bite without guilt. Remember, you control your food, it does not control you. Eat as much as you need, when you need it, not as much as you want whenever you want it. There is a difference. Stop grounding yourself from food. Give yourself permission to eat if you are hungry, even if it has only been an hour since your last meal. Just chalk it up to a high metabolism day. Fuel that flame, ladies and gentlemen!

Mapping Your Route

The Menus

"While we are on the subject of menus, Thanksgiving is just around the corner. I have now lost 23½ inches! I can't believe I'm so addicted to the tape measure! This year I fear Thanksgiving. I worry if the family will notice my shrinking state. If they ask me if I am losing weight, I will say NO!' To say yes, in their minds, would mean I am on a diet and there certainly will be disapproval at every bite of food I put into my mouth. I can not take any more disapproval," Jan says.

Breakfasts

The most important meal of the day is breakfast. Get that metabolism going!

WARNING: Read those labels. For example, English muffins can range from 130 calories up to 240 calories, and from 1 to 3 grams or more of fat! Vary the flavors of the breads you buy. You can find some wonderful fruit breads and fruit muffins or bagels!

Please note: We do not always use milk on hot cereal. Sometimes we prefer applesauce or fresh fruit. If you like milk or prefer to use a fat-free creamer, you will need to adjust your protein and/or carbohydrate percentages accordingly. For example, any time you see cottage cheese listed, you might want to replace some of that with your milk, however, cottage cheese does contain a lot more protein and less carbohydrate than milk.

The following are examples of how we eat. Of course, we modify traditional versions to reduce sugar and fat content. Some recipes, indicated by a *, are provided in a later chapter.

169

- One Egg "McMel" Muffin with low-fat or nonfat cheese and turkey ham, fruit, coffee or tea. (Use nonfat creamer and artificial sweetener if you desire)
- One English muffin, one bagel, two slices whole-wheat toast or two crumpets, toasted with two tablespoons of fat-free cream cheese, and if you like, topped with some unsweetened spread or applesauce. One cup nonfat or 1% cottage cheese, one serving of fresh fruit, coffee or tea.
- Coffee or tea, one to one and one-half servings of hot or cold cereal, one cup nonfat milk, one serving fresh fruit, one slice of toast or one-half bagel or English muffin topped with nonfat cream cheese.
- Coffee or tea, one serving of fruit, one English muffin topped with one-half cup water-packed tuna mixed with some fat-free mayonnaise. For an added treat, stick it under the broiler with some soy or almond based, cheddar or mozzarella cheese! If fish is not your fancy, have a real treat once in a while. On one-half of the muffin spread one tablespoon of fat-free cream cheese and one to one and one-half teaspoons of natural peanut butter. The cream cheese lets you use less peanut butter but you get all of the peanut butter taste and texture. Go for the chunky! Just don't do this more than once or twice a week unless you are really good at managing your daily fat grams!
- Veggie cheese omelet, two bread servings, one fruit serving, coffee or tea.
- Four multi-grain pancakes* topped with cinnamon apple sauce, one-half cup fat-free or 1% cottage cheese or one-half container of fruit yogurt, coffee or tea.
- Two bread servings, one container fruit yogurt (Try using yogurt as a spread for bread!), one serving of fruit, coffee or tea.
- Two thick slices of French toast, one-half cup nonfat or low-fat cottage cheese or one-half container of fruit yogurt, one serving of fruit, coffee or tea.
- Multi-grain waffles topped with fresh fruit and fat-free whipped topping, two ounces low-fat or fat-free turkey sausage or turkey ham, or one serving vegetarian breakfast sausage, coffee or tea.
- One container fruit yogurt mixed with one-half cup whole-grain cold cereal (without added fat or sugar), one serving fruit, coffee or tea.

- Fat-free/fruit sweetened muffins, two scrambled eggs (egg substitute), one serving of fruit, coffee or tea.
- Ham and cheese omelet or ham and scrambled eggs substitute (Use turkey ham and low-fat or nonfat cheese), one serving of bread, one fat-free frozen hash brown patty, one serving of fruit, coffee or tea.
- Two scrambled eggs, two low-fat sausage links, one pear, one cinnamon raisin English muffin.
- "Cereal" of leftover brown rice with cinnamon and sugar substitute, fruit, fruit yogurt, coffee or tea.

Lunches:

Melonie usually eats lunch on the run. When she has time to cook, she often eats one of the dinner menus or leftovers from the night before. Jan either packs her lunch or goes to a nearby deli, and orders her food as *she* wants it.

- Turkey sandwich on two slices whole-wheat bread, fat-free mayo, garden salad with fat-free dressing, hot vegetables or a piece of fruit or a toaster pastry (low-fat, fruit, sweetened).
- Tuna-salad sandwich on pita bread (water-pack tuna and fat-free mayonnaise), vegetables or a green salad, one cookie (low-fat, fruit juice, sweetened) or one-half cup frozen yogurt.
- Humus, on pita bread, and some fruit.
- Two cups black bean and rice soup, fruit or green salad.
- Grilled, low-fat cheese sandwich* on whole-wheat bread, hot veggies.
- Peanut butter and jelly sandwich on a plain bagel.
- One and one-half cup of Raisin Bran with one cup nonfat milk, fruit.
- One serving of pasta with tomato sauce, one slice of garlic bread, green salad.
- One veggie pizza,* fruit
- One hot dog or burger, fruit
- One omelet with veggies or cheese (sometimes both), two slices of toast or two bread servings, fruit.
- One cup nonfat or 1% cottage cheese, two fruits, one bread or a cookie.
- Nachos, green salad, fruit

    Or, most any repeat of one of the breakfast menus or dinner menus.

Dinners

You can be as adventurous or mundane as you like. Melonie likes to experiment with ethnic foods.

- Turkey or chicken fajitas,* green salad, fruit.
- Sautéed or broiled cod or tuna steak (or other low-fat seafood) with prepared shiitaki mushroom sauce, one cup brown and wild rice with onions and shiitake mushrooms, Caesar salad,* one slice of garlic bread, fruit.
- Shrimp Caesar salad, one serving of cornbread, fruit.
- Chicken, turkey, shrimp or vegetarian curry,* one cup brown rice or brown basmati rice, garden salad or hot vegetable, fruit.
- "Fried" chicken, one cup rice or one baked potato or one serving of pasta with fat-free toppings of choice, Caesar* or garden salad, one serving of bread, fruit.
- Two soft tacos with salsa and sour cream,* vegetarian refried beans with cheese, veggies or salad, fruit.
- One serving pasta (two ounces dry) with alfredo or tomato sauce, two slices garlic bread, Caesar salad,* fruit yogurt.
- Noodles with three-cheese casserole, hot veggies, green salad, fruit.
- Stir-fried Thai veggies, brown rice or soba noodles, fruit, pudding or frozen yogurt.
- Two veggie pizzas,* green salad, fruit.
- Shrimp jambalya, hot veggies, fruit.
- Vegetarian chili with cheese, one tortilla, green salad, fruit.
- Vegetarian stew with fennel and bell peppers, brown rice, one slice French bread, fruit.
- Cheeseburger,* green salad, fruit.
- Swedish meatballs,* noodles, green salad, veggies, fruit.
- Scalloped potatoes with ham, hot veggies, green salad, fruit.
- One serving of turkey or chicken breast, with fat-free or low-fat sauce (if desired), mashed potatoes and fat-free gravy or oven fries or baked potato or rice or pasta or stuffing, hot veggies, fruit.
- Cabbage au gratin,* salad, two bread servings, fruit.
- Meatloaf,* baked potato with cheddar cheese, hot veggies, green salad, lemon pie.
- Macaroni and cheese,* green salad, veggies, fruit.
- Tuna-noodle casserole, green salad, hot veggies, fruit.
- Curried rice with chicken salad, hot or cold veggies, fresh fruit, frozen yogurt.
- Grilled chicken or turkey Caesar, two slices garlic bread, fruit, fudge brownies.*

Snacks

Most often these should be complex carbohydrates, or occasionally a fruit yogurt or some frozen yogurt, or some cold cereal with fruit and milk, or a low-fat, juice-sweetened toaster pastry or healthy granola bar, or some pretzels and fruit. If you get full before you eat your fruit at meal time, have your fruit for a snack. Fruit should be complemented with a serving of bread, to help stabilize the rise in blood sugar from the fruit. If you are not hungry, it is OK to skip a snack.

Helpful hints

Just balance your meals among the food groups, making sure you keep it at approximately 10–30 percent protein, nor more than 30 percent fat (for BodyLogic freshmen!) and the balance in complex carbohydrate. For example, if you choose a meal of stir-fry veggies over rice, you might want to have a fruit yogurt, pudding or frozen yogurt for desert to make sure you get your protein.

The menus provided are the way *we* eat. We consume very little pork or red meat. Depending on what time of day your activity break happens, plan to have a meal higher in complex carbohydrates an hour or so before you get moving. You need to adapt your favorite recipes to the way *you* eat. Eating pork or red meat is fine as long as the total fat grams for the meal remain less than 30 percent. Veggies and fruit are not required at every meal. Melonie will take inventory of her food for the day after her noon meal. If she finds she is lacking in any of the food groups, she structures the remainder of her snacks and evening meal to make sure she eats at least the minimum number of servings from each food group.

No one is perfect. Some days you may crave protein and lack in your fruits and veggies. Other days, especially during the hot summer months, you may go several days without meeting your protein requirements. Just evaluate what you eat frequently so you can get your food plan back on track. For example, if it's 100 degrees outside, we might eat a fruit plate with fruit yogurt and a slice of bread for one or several meals. While a bit too low in fat, at least it provides complex carbos and protein. You should not try to go below 10 percent of calories from fat, but if you do, your body probably won't notice if this only happens for a few days. Your body will notice if you do not get adequate protein or complex carbohydrates. You can never have too many veggies (unless they are potatoes, peas or corn, which we consider to be more simple carbohydrate rather than vegetables).

For every decrease of one fat gram you get to eat two extra protein or complex carbo grams for the same number of calories. If you are getting hungry any more often than every two and one half to three hours on a daily basis, you may need to up your calories a bit (or reevaluate your fat intake and make sure it is at least 10 percent). Increase those calories by adding complex carbohydrates like whole grains and fruits. If your meal plans usually carry you two and one half to three hours, but occasionally you have a day where you feel starving all of the time, go ahead and eat more, starting with extra servings of complex carbos. Eat when you are really hungry, not by the clock. Eat six times a day if you need to. Eat balanced meals. Eat what you like with healthy substitutions where needed.

Finally, *never ever* say to yourself, "I was bad with my food today." Or, "I am a bad person because I had that piece of cheesecake." Those messages only serve to facilitate the diet mentality. That mentality will not foster a healthy lifelong change in eating habits. Instead say, "That piece of cheesecake really satisfied my craving. I'll cut back a few fat grams each day for the next two to three days." Or, "My foodstyle has been out of balance for a week because I was staying with friends and was not able to choose my food as I would have liked. I also was not as active as usual. I really enjoyed my visit, but it is good to be home and back in my routine. I'll start up where I left off, and maybe throw in a couple of after-dinner walks this week." Give yourself permission to be human. Just don't let being human on occasion become a routine. Think about how much better you feel now, how much more energy and strength you have. Maybe you had fewer illnesses last winter, and you are sleeping better too! Let these thoughts be your motivation to continue with a healthier lifestyle. Again, it's not necessarily about losing weight, though that is a nice benefit of improving your lifestyle. You can improve your health, be more fit and still be overfat. That's one big improvement over being ill, out of breath, fatigued and overfat, too!

> *Your positive self statement for today: "I do not care what others think of me. In my eyes, their disapproval only means a lack of knowledge. I*

am not committing to this lifestyle change to gain approval from anyone but myself. I will not be my own worse enemy. I will proudly acknowledge to the world that I am indeed an incredible shrinking person! I love the changes that I see in the mirror! I love the changes in my soul! I love myself!"

Detours

Sample Menu Make-overs

Before we dive into the recipes, lets have a look-see at how some very simple, well-planned substitutions can turn a high fat, low-nutrition meal into something your body will smile about!

When we first started our lifestyle changes, we began to keep food diaries as a reference point. We have provided you with a one-day sample of what our meals looked like before and after Body-Logic worked its magic. Keep in mind, Mel no longer needs to consume as many calories as are in the majority of these meals, but the calorie counts are quite typical for Jan these days. This is simply a learning tool. Again, we do not expect you to eat exactly like we do. The focus here is to learn what a balanced meal looks like, and how simple it is to make a few healthy substitutions to help you achieve that balance. When doctors are in medical school, they learn to read X-rays by studying "healthy" films. Once they know what "healthy" looks like, they can more easily recognize what "unhealthy" looks like. We will take the same approach here. OK students (and future BodyLogic specialists)—here we go!

Unhealthy	Healthy
2 scrambled eggs with butter	2 scrambled "egg substitute"
2 Tbsp. Half & Half,	eggs or eggs (whites only) with
2 English muffins	2 Tbsp. skim milk (cooked
4 Tbsp. regular cream cheese	using spray oil).
	2 English muffins
	4 Tbsp. fat-free cream cheese
	3 oz. fat-free turkey sausage
	1 peach

1 cup oatmeal (unflavored)
¾ cup skim milk

Here're the numbers!

Calories:	750			Calories:	741	
Protein:	29	(16%)		Protein:	55	(32%)
Carb:	54	(31%)		Carb:	105	(63%)
Fat:	**43**	**(53%)**		**Fat:**	**4**	**(5%)**

The redo is within spitting distance as far as calories go. We added a serving of fruit and a serving of dairy to balance the meal according to food groups. But look at the big picture! You get nearly twice as much food just by eliminating the majority of the fat! How could you be hungry after consuming the "healthy" meal? Yes, we admit it's a bit low in fat. Not to worry. You can make up that fat later in the day! Now lets play with lunch a bit:

Unhealthy	Healthy
3 beef hot dogs	3 turkey hot dogs
3 hot dog buns	3 hot dog buns
1 apple	1 apple
	small green salad
	1 low-fat, fruit-sweetened
	oatmeal raisin cookie
	1 cup 1% milk

Here're the numbers!

Calories	789			Calories:	853	
Protein	4	(12%)		Protein·	48	(23%)
Carb:	66	(35%)		Carb:	136	(67%)
Fat	**45**	**(53%)**		**Fat:**	**10**	**(10%)**

Look how much more food you get for just a few more calories! Even more impressive, look at the reduction in fat grams and the balance achieved with the make-over! Something from each food group, and "something sweet for the sweet."

Original	Make-over
2 cups macaroni and cheese	3 cups Mel's Smacaroni and cheese
2 cups frozen mixed veggies with margarine	3 cups frozen mixed veggies butter substitute
1 pint of Rocky Road ice cream	4 oz. turkey breast
(Yes, we used to eat like this!)	1 pint fat-free frozen yogurt

Here're the numbers:

Calories:	2035		Calories:	2017	
Protein:	55	(10%)	Protein:	151	(30%)
Carb:	197	(39%)	Carb:	305	(62%)
Fat:	**113**	**(51%)**	**Fat:**	**8**	**(8%)**

Pretty amazing huh? More than one and one half times more food for a skosh fewer calories, and look at that fat gram count!

How about a typical snack:

Unhealthy	Healthy
1 small bag potato chips	1 small bag of pretzels
1 bran muffin with raisins	1 bagel with 2 Tbsp. reduced-fat peanut butter
1 banana	1 banana

Here're the numbers:

Unhealthy			Healthy		
Calories	375		Calories:	670	
Protein	6	(6%)	Protein:	19	(11%)
Carb:	59	(62%)	Carb:	115	(70%)
Fat	**13**	**(32%)**	**Fat:**	**14**	**(19%)**

OK. You got us this time. The snacks are not perfectly balanced. But we did tell you the fat grams would be made up later in the day! Yes, there are a lot more calories in the "healthy" snack. Likely, if you have been eating meals like those listed as "unhealthy," you might not have been getting enough calories, nor the right kind of calories. If you are hungry, like we typically are every three hours, you eat more food as long as that food is high octane!

Have we made our point yet? It's not so much the *quantity* of food, but the *quality* of the food that counts! How far would your car run if you put whisky or rubbing alcohol in the tank instead of premium unleaded gasoline? Enough said.

All it takes is just a few simple substitutions in what food you buy, and a few alterations in the way you typically prepare your food. It's almost like magic, it's so simple! Look at the next chapter, on recipes, for lots of ideas on how you can modify your favorite meals, mostly made with products you would typically find at your local grocery store. Get creative. Challenge yourself. Amaze yourself. Just remember, the first revision of any recipe may not be perfect, and in fact, may not be fit for the cat to eat. But with each mistake you make, you learn. We hope we have paved the way so that your mistakes are few, and your successes are many!

Pleasurable Side Trips

Recipe Re-Do's

These are samples. They are provided to show you ways you can adapt your favorite menus to make them healthy, tasty, and often better than the original. In the beginning, you will notice the reduced fat, but in time, you won't think twice about it. Being single women, neither of us have much desire or time for cooking. We demand easy, fast, balanced meals that taste great and for the most part don't require a special trip to the store just to fix one meal. One thing you will notice is most of the recipes serve one. That's because each of us cook for one. We are tired of adapting recipes that serve eight to something that serves one. It just never comes out the same way. It's much easier to multiply a recipe by the number of servings than to try to figure out how to divide one tablespoon of something by eight! These serving sizes are good size. If you can only have a tiny bit of something you can barely see, why bother?

Notes:

Aspartame is the main ingredient in NutraSweet and similar sweeteners. Substitute your preferred sweetener. Spray oil refers to products such as PAM.

We are both "pitch-and-throw" cooks. We seldom measure anything! We have tried to estimate the ingredient quantities as closely as possible, but please forgive us if things don't always go just perfectly when you make the recipes. Part of the fun of this is adapting things to your own liking, so feel free to substitute, pitch and throw to your heart's content, as long as the result is low fat!

Salad dressings

Mel's "Maybe Creamy Caesar Dressing"

¼ cup Angostura soy or teriyaki sauce
¼ cup fresh or regular strength bottled lemon juice
2–3 cloves of fresh garlic or a comparable amount of crushed garlic in the jar
¼ cup nonfat sour cream or mayonnaise (optional)
1 Tbsp. of fat-free Parmesan, if desired
Fresh-ground pepper to taste
Throw it in the blender until smooth, and store in the fridge. It keeps well. Just give a quick stir before using.

Here're the numbers. Talk about drama!
Serving size: 2 Tbsp.

Mel's "Maybe Creamy Caesar"			Bottled Caesar dressing		
Calories:	12		Calories:	158	
Protein:	0		Protein:	0	
Carb:	3	(100%)	Carb:	0	
Fat:	**0**	**(0%)**	**Fat:**	**17**	**(100%)**

Mel's "Honey of a Dijon"

This one's great because there is no added sugar, and it literally takes about one minute to fix!
About ⅓ cup bottled fat-free Caesar dressing
About 1 tsp. Dijon mustard
About 1 packet of aspartame (the sweetness of 1 tsp. sugar)
Mix it all up. Adjust the ingredients to your taste. The numbers are insignificant, maybe 30 calories per serving.

Mel's Poppy Seed Dressing:

Do the same as with the Honey Dijon, only substitute poppy seeds for the Dijon mustard. It doesn't get much easier than that.

Bread and Breakfast

Mel's "Garlic Breath"

Find a good Italian bread without fat listed in the ingredients. Cut into one to one-and-one-half-inch slices. Spray lightly with spray oil or brush *very* lightly with olive oil. Thinly spread with crushed garlic or give a light sprinkle of garlic powder. Finish with a light grinding of sea salt if desired. Stick it under the broiler until golden. For variety, and to get extra protein if needed, when nearly done top with some fat-free Parmesan or some grated nonfat or low-fat cheese alternative (Melonie likes the soy- or almond-based ones for their flavor and meltability.) For added variety, substitute whole wheat pita bread for each serving and prepare it the same way.

Here are the numbers for a two-ounce slice, using spray oil for Mel's version:

Mel's Garlic Bread:			Traditional Garlic Bread		
Calories:	140		Calories:	159	
Protein:	4	(12%)	Protein:	3	(7%)
Carb:	26	(82%)	Carb:	22	(58%)
Fat:	**1**	**(6%)**	**Fat:**	**6**	**(35%)**

Mel's "10-Grain Emerald City Muffins"

Yield: About 7

Serving size: It's up to you. These are true guilt-free comfort food! (For the sake of the numbers, we will call one serving one muffin.)

Prep time: 5 minutes

Baking time: 20 minutes

Love muffins? Ever try to make a low-fat or fat-free muffin and end up with a brick? Even some of the best recipes out there for "low-fat muffins" have an average of 5–6 fat grams per serving, which calculates to as much as 24 percent fat for just one little muffin! I love muffins. I also hate the "fat-free" ones in the store that are full of sugar and have more calories than the original version. How could I lower the fat, and keep the flavor and texture of the real thing? And of course it must be moist! Don't know what it is about 90 degree weather that sparks the baking bug. "She must be crazy!" Anyone who knows me will attest to that fact! Then it hit me, right smack dab in the face. What other food has the closest texture to muffins? Pancakes! Here's what I came up with on that hot summer day. This is another one of those great recipes that you can change to your heart's content. Use them for dinner instead of bread (throw some crushed garlic, onion powder, dill, nonfat soy cheese, etc. into the mix), use them for breakfast (toss in two or three packets of aspartame, add some fresh, mashed banana, maybe some blueberries, even mix in some cocoa into the dry ingredients, etc. before baking). I like mine plain so I can put most anything on them. The recipe as is produces a muffin that is really not sweet at all, so adjust the sweetness as you like it! This way I can use one batch all day long. You won't believe this one:

In a blender or a mixing bowl, combine:
¼ cup low-fat (1–2%) cottage cheese or plain nonfat yogurt
1 tsp. butter substitute sprinkles
½ cup water
1½ tsp. powdered buttermilk
¼ cup fat-free egg substitute
2 Tbsp. skim milk
Blend the whole mess in the blender or using a hand mixer.

In another small bowl (or be lazy and use a large measuring cup), mix together with a fork:
1 cup 10-grain pancake mix (1 fat gram per serving please)
½ tsp. baking powder

Dump the dry stuff into the wet stuff and quickly mix well with a fork. Do not overmix.

Spritz some regular-size muffin tins with spray oil (unless you have good nonstick ones, then you can eliminate the spray oil). Fill the tins two-thirds to three-fourths full with the batter. If there are any empty sections, put some water in them to keep the heat distribution even and to add moisture. I also stick a small dish of water in the oven for extra moisture.

Bake at 400 degrees for twenty minutes or until they feel done when touched, golden on the top, or until a toothpick inserted in the center comes out clean. Do not overbake. Allow to cool for ten minutes or so before removing from the tins. Eat them up any way you want. Pour on some nonfat margarine substitute (I like the spray kind but I pour it on everything!), jam, applesauce, fruit yogurt, nonfat cream cheese, nonfat gravy, anything nonfat that you want.

Here're the numbers:

Mel's 10-Grain Emerald City Muffins			Traditional Muffins		
Each one contains:					
Calories:	46		Calories:	140	
Protein:	4	(35%)	Protein:	3	(9%)
Carb:	7	(63%)	Carb:	19	(58%)
Fat:	**.5**	**(2%)**	**Fat:**	**5**	**(33%)**

"If It Walks Like a Duck...It Must Be Mel's Biscuits!"

Yield: It depends on the size (I get six).
Serving size is one biscuit
Prep time: 5 minutes
Baking time: 10–12 minutes
Eating time: About 30 seconds!

OK. So the muffin recipe got me to thinking. If I can make moist, fluffy muffins that taste great and are essentially fat and sugar free, why not biscuits? OK. So I lied. The muffin recipe was my first attempt at biscuits! Remember what I said about your first try at modifying any recipe may not give you the result you want? Forgot to mention that sometimes you end up with something better than you had planned in the first place! Even the best "low-fat" biscuit recipes have up to 4 fat grams or more per serving—that's 25 percent calories from fat! For just one. I don't know about you but I feel deprived if I can eat only one of anything. Which would you rather have, a credit card limit of $100 or $1,000? So I heated up the oven again on that same hot summer day and here's what happened.

(Read the entire recipe first for some valuable helpful hints!)
In a medium bowl, mix together with a fork:
¼ cup sifted unbleached white flour
¾ cup sifted cake flour
1 tsp. butter flavor sprinkles
¼ tsp. salt
¼ tsp. baking soda
¾ tsp. baking powder
(If you like a sweeter biscuit, add a half packet of aspartame or a teaspoon of sugar)
In a measuring cup, mix about one-half cup buttermilk made from

one and one-half tablespoons powdered buttermilk (nonfat) and one-half cup water.

To the flour mixture, add a heaping one-fourth cup of low-fat cottage cheese (substitute plain nonfat yogurt if you prefer), about one-third at a time and cut it in with a fork. Keep cutting in and adding the cottage cheese until the mixture looks like mostly peas with some flour leftovers. Try not to mix it too much. Make a well in the center. Add one-fourth cup of the buttermilk mixture and stir gently just until it forms a very soft, slightly sticky ball. Once the initial stirring is done, use your fingers to incorporate the rest of the flour. When it's just right, you should have a slightly sticky ball similar to the feel of a moist bread dough. Lightly spritz a muffin tin with some spray oil. Hey, it's not that I am lazy, even though I am. You know as well as I any pastry dough should be handled as little as possible to keep it tender. You can roll it out and cut it up like old-fashioned biscuits, but it will come out tough. Form the dough into balls about the size of golf balls and lightly press one into each muffin tin section. Brush with some of the buttermilk and bake at 425 degrees (set a small dish of water in the oven during preheating and while baking for extra moisture) for ten minutes. They may not be brown. Do not overbake! If these come out kind of like little sponges, you baked them too long, you handled them too much or you did not use enough liquid in the dough. Keep the dough so sticky you can barely form it into balls. You can spoon the dough into the tins instead to further reduce how much you handle it. This recipe takes a bit of practice, but it's well worth it! Use them any way you would traditional muffins. Enjoy! (I finally satisfied that biscuit craving!)

Here're the numbers:

Mel's "Ducky" Biscuits 1 26-gram biscuit			Traditional Biscuits 1 26-gram biscuit		
Calories:	66		Calories:	98	
Protein:	3	(21%)	Protein:	1	(4%)
Carb:	12	(79%)	Carb:	12	(59%)
Fat:	**0**	**(ZILCH!)**	**Fat:**	**4**	**(37%)**

Cornbread (makes 12 servings)

In a medium bowl, combine:
1 cup unbleached white flour
1 cup pure ground cornmeal
1 Tbsp. baking powder
1½ tsp. salt

In another medium bowl, combine:
½ cup unsweetened applesauce
⅓ cup fat-free mayo
¼ cup egg substitute
1 cup skim milk or nonfat buttermilk

Add the wet mixture to the dry, and mix just until blended. One secret of fat-free baking is not to overmix. This will make the finished product tough!

If you like a sweeter cornbread, you can add six packets or six teaspoons of aspartame to the dry ingredients, *or* one-fourth cup of Barley Malt or fruit-based sweetener to the wet ingredients. If using "wet" sweeteners, adjust the skim milk down so you get the right thickness to the batter. The batter should be thick yet still pourable.

Spread into an 8 x 8 inch baking pan lined with parchment or lightly sprayed with spray oil. Bake twenty-five to thirty minutes at 400 degrees, or just until a toothpick placed in the center comes out clean. Let cool five to ten minutes before serving. Top with some I Can't Believe It's Not Butter spray or for a special, occasional treat, a bit of honey!

This cornbread is *very* moist!

Here are the numbers:

Mel's Cornbread			Traditional Cornbread		
Per recipe or 1 serving:					
Calories:	116		Calories:	190	
Protein:	4	(11%)	Protein:	4	(9%)
Carb:	30	(89%)	Carb:	27	(62%)
Fat:	**0**	**(ZILCH!)**	**Fat:**	**6**	**(29%)**

If you must have sugar, replace the one-half cup applesauce with one-fourth cup sugar. This will add 15 calories and 3 carbohydrates per serving.

French Toast

2 slices of good Italian bread, with no fat added (1–1½ inch slices, about 2 oz.

Mix together:

¼ cup egg substitute

¼–½ cup skim milk

artificial sweetener to taste

cinnamon to taste

Soak the bread in the egg mixture on both sides. This may take a while if the bread is not very fresh. Heat up a nonstick griddle or fry pan and give it a light dusting of spray oil. Add the bread to the pan and cook over medium heat until golden, about three-to-five minutes per side. Don't get the pan too hot or the bread will be burnt on the outside and gooey on the inside! Top with fresh fruit, applesauce, fruit yogurt, fruit spread or artificially sweetened syrup.

Here's a great idea for breakfast on the run. Cut the bread into sticks before you egg and grill it. You have your own healthy version of fast-food French toast sticks!

And the numbers are:

Mel's French Toast:			Fast-Food Version:		
Calories:	195		Calories:	500	
Protein:	13	(30%)	Protein:	4	(3%)
Carb:	29	(70%)	Carb:	60	(48%)
Fat:	**0**	**ZERO**	**Fat**	**27**	**(49%)**

Pancakes

serves: 1

Mix together in a medium bowl JUST UNTIL BLENDED:

½ cup multi-grain pancake and waffle mix (look in the natural-food section or specialty flour section to find a brand with 1 fat gram per serving as packaged)

¼ cup egg substitute

¼ cup unsweetened applesauce

Add skim milk or water to desired thickness.

For added variety, toss in some fresh or frozen berries, or some fresh finely chopped banana or apple. Cook over medium heat using a nonstick fry pan or griddle with a light touch of spray oil. Top with what you like. See the French toast recipe for ideas.

Here are the numbers: (About four cakes / 240 grams total)

Mel's Pancakes:			Traditional Pancakes:		
Calories:	257		Calories:	529	
Protein:	16	(26%)	Protein:	16	(12%)
Carb:	43	(71%)	Carb:	73	(57%)
Fat:	**1**	**(3%)**	**Fat:**	**18**	**(31%)**

For waffles: Use the same recipe. You can add in some stiffly beaten egg white. The batter should be quite thick. Use a nonstick waffle maker or coat a traditional waffle iron with some spray oil. Top with a mound of fresh berries and fat-free whipped topping. Enjoy it in bed! Who needs to go out for brunch!

Soups

Jan's "Foggy" Soup

Just in case you have never been to the Northwest in the fall and winter months, we describe the fog as, "thick as pea soup." Here's Jan's version. We promise it won't reduce your visibility one bit, unless the amount of visible "stuff" is on your body!

Stick it in the crockpot in the morning, finish it off in the evening, and you have a heartwarming, heart-healthy first course or main meal!

Serves: 8
Prep time: 15 minutes
Cooking time: 4–8 hours, unsupervised

Ingredients:
1 small package of dried split peas, rinsed and sorted through
1 huge onion, chopped
¾ small bag or a whole bag of baby carrots, sliced
8 cups of water
1½ lbs. turkey ham, cut to desired size
1–2 tsp. marjoram, as much as desired
garlic powder or fresh garlic to taste
black pepper to taste

Dump everything except the carrots into the crockpot. If you will be out all day, set it on low. If you will be around, you can use low or high. Whatever you want to do is fine!

About one hour before the end of the cooking time, throw in the carrots. Continue cooking just until the carrots are done. Stir occasionally if you are around to think about it!

Here are the numbers:

Jan's "Foggy" Soup			Traditional Soup with Ham		
Calories:	402		Calories:	582	
Protein:	33	(33%)	Protein:	38	(26%)
Carb:	56	(58%)	Carb:	56	(39%)
Fat:	**4**	**(9%)**	**Fat:**	**22**	**(35%)**

Want to cut those numbers even more? Use ¾ lb. turkey ham and add some Liquid Smoke flavoring to taste. The protein and fat counts will be cut in half. Want to be totally obsessive compulsive? Substitute 4–6 ounces of fat-free turkey sausage and a splash of Liquid Smoke for the turkey ham. How does one little old fat gram grab you?

Jan's "Everything But The Kitchen Sink, Almost" Soup

Serves: 8
Prep time: 20 minutes
Cooking time: About an hour, unsupervised
Ingredients:
1 46-oz. can tomato or V8 juice (Use reduced-sodium variety)
2 cup water
2 cup chopped carrots
2 cup shredded cabbage
2 cup green beans (fresh, frozen or canned)
2 cup zucchini, sliced
1 small head of cauliflower broken into small pieces
1 medium onion, chopped
1 tablespoon dried basil, crushed
½ tablespoon garlic powder
½ tablespoon pepper

Put everything into a large pot and simmer until the veggies are tender crisp, or as desired. Serve in pretty soup bowls, with a sprinkling of fat-free Parmesan cheese on top.

The numbers are not even worth mentioning. Trust us, it's fat-free! You can do whatever you want with this soup. Add potatoes, carrots, pinto beans, cauliflower, broccoli, mushrooms, everything but the kitchen sink (and fat of course).

In case you are curious, the numbers for the traditional version are also hardly worth mentioning. But we think you will agree our version tastes much better than something out of a can!

Veggies

Mel's Zucchini Stir-Fry

Serves: 1
Prep time: 5 minutes max
Cooking time: 10–15 minutes
Ingredients:
1 small zucchini
1 small vine-ripened tomato
¼ cup fat-free pasta sauce
crushed garlic
salt, pepper and red pepper flakes to taste

This is too simple. Slice up the zucchini and throw it in a nonstick pan, lightly coated with spray oil. Cook it on medium heat. When the zucchini is about half done (don't overcook) throw in the garlic, tomatoes, pasta sauce and seasoning. Continue cooking and stir occasionally. When the zucchini is done, plate it up and sprinkle with some fat-free, herb-blend Parmesan cheese.

The numbers? About 40 calories, 1 gram of protein and 9 grams of carbohydrates. No fat here!

Mel's "I'm a cooked-cabbage convert!" Cabbage Au Gratin

Serves: 2
Prep time: about 20 minutes
Baking time: about 30–40 minutes

This one is guaranteed to turn a cooked-cabbage hater into a cooked-cabbage lover. I was introduced to the original version in a gourmet foods class in college. Of the thirty students in the class, not one continued to hate cooked cabbage after trying it. My version has much less fat, but tastes just as good!

Ingredients:
½ head fresh green cabbage
6 oz. nonfat soy cheese (cheddar, or mozzarella, or a mixture!)
1 can low-fat, reduced-sodium cream of chicken, or cream of mushroom soup
⅓ cup or so of skim milk
1 chicken bullion cube
fat-free saltine cracker or bread crumbs
fresh-ground pepper

Wash and trim the cabbage and separate the leaves. Preheat the oven to 350 degrees. Bring a large pot of salted water to the boil. Throw in the cabbage and cook just for a couple of minutes, until it is bright green and barely tender crisp. Immediately drain and rinse with cold water to stop the cooking. Don't overcook the cabbage. While the cabbage is cooling some, throw the soup into a saucepan and mix in enough skim milk to make the whole thing the consistency of a moderately thick white sauce. You want it moist and creamy but not runny. Crush the bullion cube inside a plastic bag, using a hammer or some such thing! Sprinkle the bullion over the soup mixture and heat up the whole thing just until it is warm. Season with pepper to taste. While that is heating, grate up the cheese. Reserve about one-third cup or so, and throw the rest into the soup mixture. Stir until the cheese is melted. If the mixture seems too thick, add more milk or some water. Set the sauce aside. Lightly spritz a small baking dish (at least two inches deep) with some spray oil. Place a layer of cabbage in the bottom, then a layer of the soup mixture, then a layer of cabbage. Continue layering, ending with the soup mixture on top. Sprinkle the reserved cheese over the top, then scatter the bread or cracker crumbs (about one-eighth cup). Bake at 350 until heated through, about thirty to forty minutes. About twenty minutes into the baking, cover with foil to preserve moisture. This prevents the cheese on the top from turning into a rock. (Spray the foil with a bit of spray oil to prevent the cheese from sticking to it.)

Let the whole mess cool for ten minutes or so and serve it up. This one is great with fish or chicken, or pork roast if you are so inclined! Another variation, in place of the soup and milk mixture, is to make a white sauce using evaporated skim milk, butter spray (poured in), and thickened with a mixture of flour or cornstarch and water. Continue fixing it the same way. Don't forget the bullion cube, as this is the magic ingredient.

Here're the numbers (made with soup):

Mel's Cabbage Au Gratin			Traditional Version		
Calories:	283		Calories:	550	
Protein:	26	(38%)	Protein:	21	(15%)
Carb:	37	(56%)	Carb:	25	(20%)
Fat:	**2**	**(6%)**	**Fat:**	**39**	**(65%)**

Main Dishes/Entrees

Jan's "Boobs" (chicken, that is!)

This is truly an original, one-of-a-kind recipe. Got twenty minutes? You have a gourmet feast! Ever tried to fix boneless, skinless chicken breasts and end up with a version similar to what your grandmother wore? (You know, dry and shriveled up!) This chicken is so moist, it's beyond belief! Here it goes:

Serves: 1

Serving size: 3 ounces

Prep time: 1–2 minutes

Cooking time: 15–20 minutes

Clean and trim the boobs of all fat. Put them in a large skillet. Sprinkle with a teaspoon of dried basil or up to a tablespoon of fresh basil. Add as much as you like. Experiment with different herbs or even garlic powder or fresh garlic cloves! Cover the boobs with water. Bring to a slow boil, reduce the heat and simmer uncovered fifteen to twenty minutes or until done. Turn at least once. Serve with rice, smashed spuds, pasta or whatever you like, and don't forget a big plate of veggies to go with it!

Here're the numbers (for one-half breast, about three ounces):

Jan's "Boobs"			Traditional Sautéed Chicken		
Calories:	141		Calories:	213	
Protein:	26	(81%)	Protein:	31	(66%)
Carb:	0		Carb:	0	
Fat:	**3**	**(19%)**	**Fat:**	**8**	**(34%)**

Mel's "Gobble 'Em Up Quarter Pounder"

Serves: 1

Prep time: 1 minute

Cooking time: About 5 minutes

Ingredients:

1 (4 oz.) extra-lean ground turkey patty

garlic powder to taste

salt and pepper to taste

1 whole-wheat hamburger bun

A couple thin slices of sweet onion, cut into large pieces

bottled barbecue sauce or steak sauce to taste (watch the fat content!)

Toast the bun under the broiler if you like it that way. Just use a spritz of spray oil. Meanwhile, heat up a nonstick griddle or fry pan over medium low heat. Season the patty with salt, pepper and garlic powder to taste. Put the patty in the pan and scatter the onions around the sides. When the patty is cooked about half way, flip it over. Give the onions a stir at the same time. (Don't forget the bun under the broiler.) When the patty is just firm to the touch, put it on the bun. Pour on the sauce and put the onions on top. Put on the lid and you have a moist, delicious burger. Don't overcook the meat or it will turn out more like a rubber chicken! For something extra special, melt some nonfat cheese over the top of the cooked meat before you add the onions and sauce. Try throwing some fresh, sliced mushrooms in with the onions. You will need a bib for this version.

Serve it up with a big green salad, fresh corn on the cob and some baked potato chips and you have one heck of a meal.

Here are the numbers:

Mel's "Gobble 'Em Up" Quarter-Pounder:			Traditional BeefBurger:		
Calories:	290		Calories:	531	
Protein:	34	(47%)	Protein:	26	(20%)
Carb:	29	(41%)	Carb:	38	(30%)
Fat:	**4**	**(12%)**	**Fat:**	**29**	**(50%)**

Mel's "Too Good To Be True Pizza"

Serves: 1

1 whole wheat or regular white pita bread

Top in the following order with:

1 packet fat-free pizza sauce

Any variety of veggies: sweet white onion, mushrooms, red or green bell pepper, broccoli and tomatoes or sundried tomatoes (not packed in oil).

2 oz. of cheese alternative

(I like a lot of red-pepper flakes sprinkled on top!)

Bake at 375 until the veggies are tender crisp and the pita bread is crispy. To get extra browning on the pita, give a light touch of spray oil before adding the pizza sauce.

To make this "unveggie," use fat-free turkey sausage, or vegetable or soy-based breakfast sausage. If you must, use a small amount of reduced-fat pepperoni, but it is high in fat and saturated fat.

You can get as creative as you like. Try some 97 percent fat-free turkey strips or a bit of chicken breast, some pineapple, some turkey ham instead of Canadian bacon. The possibilities are endless!

Here are the numbers:

Mel's Pizza:			Traditional Veggie Pizza:		
(1 pizza)			(2 slices)		
Calories:	286		Calories:	296	
Protein:	18	(29%)	Protein:	13	(18%)
Carb:	39	(65%)	Carb:	34	(48%)
Fat:	**2**	**(6%)**	**Fat:**	**11**	**(34%)**

Mel's Seattle Sunshine Meatloaf

First, if you don't live in the Northwest, Seattle Sunshine is also re-ferred to as liquid sunshine (rain). Ever try turkey meatloaf? Was your first (and likely only) attempt to simply substitute ground turkey for the ground beef? Was it the most dry, tasteless thing you ever tried to eat? I vividly remember my mother's first and only attempt at turkey meatloaf. Her intentions were good. She thought she could cut the fat by using turkey instead of beef. She was right on that concept, but neglected to realize that decreasing fat decreases flavor and moisture. To be honest with you, neither one of us (nor the cat!) could stomach that meatloaf! Keep in mind while growing up, I did eat red meat. Mom made meatloaf every Monday, and we ate meatloaf sandwiches from the leftovers (one of my favorites). So, I do have a reference point on which to compare my version with Mom's, and her's was the best "beef" meatloaf I ever tasted. It was moist, though not as moist as this version! Writing this book really sparked the cooking urge. On one of my rare quiet days, I felt fall in the air and suddenly had a meatloaf craving. So here I go again, and this one was a winner the first time around. If you are like me, the first words out of your mouth will be: "Hmm, could this be *too* moist?" And when done with the usual sized serving with all the trimmings, you might notice feel-ing a lot fuller than after the traditional beef meatloaf meal.

About 5 servings

Serving size: 3.5 ounces

Prep time: 15–45 minutes. Bake Time 60–75 minutes.

1½ cup cooked brown rice (Save time and cook ahead! It takes 45 minutes to cook!)

½ cup uncooked oatmeal (quick-cooking type, not instant)
1 cup chopped fresh mushrooms
½ cup chopped green pepper
1 small chopped onion
minced garlic to taste (I like lots, so I use about two teaspooons.)
6 oz. ground turkey
1 package of dry turkey-flavor gravy mix
¼ cup egg substitute (fat free of course)
(If it's too moist the first time, add a bit of flour the next time around.)

In a medium sauté pan, "sweat" the onions and peppers by sprinkling with a dash of salt and covering with a lid. Cook over medium heat, stirring occasionally, just until they begin to soften. Don't let them turn to mush. While the veggies are cooking, place the turkey in a medium-size mixing bowl. Stir in the garlic, then stir in the mushrooms and oatmeal. Add the egg substitute, then the rice and gravy mix, and finally the hot veggies. (Don't put the veggies directly on the egg substitute or you will end up with scrambled meatloaf!) Mix it all together very well. Add as much black pepper as you like. Save the salt to add at the table as the gravy mix has lots in it. Place the whole mess in a large (about 4½ by 9 inches) oven-safe loaf pan lightly sprayed with one of the nonstick products. Bake uncovered at 400 degrees for sixty to seventy-five minutes, or until the center feels firm when pressed and the edges are starting to get kind of crispy. (If you want spuds, throw them in at the same time the meatloaf goes in!) Allow the loaf to cool for fifteen to twenty minutes before slicing. You can always reheat in the microwave if you get wrapped up doing something, like writing a book!

For an added treat, serve with some cranberry sauce, fat-free turkey gravy or top with shiitake mushroom sauce. Serve a green salad, a baked spud with some melted nonfat cheddar cheese (nonfat sour cream and fake bacon bits if you like the works) and some hot veggies.

Don't stress over the fat content of this version. When combined as part of a well-balanced meal, you will end up with about 11 percent calories from fat from the meal which is darn good.

Here are the numbers per serving:

	Seattle Sunshine Meatloaf:		Original Turkey Loaf:		Mom's Beef Loaf:	
Calories:	556		191		239	
Protein:	12	(34%)	23	50%	18	(34%)
Carb:	16	(45%)	7	16%	6	(12%)
Fat:	**3.6**	**(21%)**	**7**	**34%**	**14**	**(54%)**

Looks can be deceiving!

OK. So you still can't get into turkey loaf. Here's a fix. Substitute beef for the turkey and beef gravy mix for the turkey gravy mix. Yes, this substitution works! Here are the numbers per serving:

Calories:	180	
Protein:	11	(26%)
Carb:	16	(39%)
Fat:	**7**	**(35%)** (Still far from home base, but a definite improvement!)

Mel's "Svedish Meatballs, and then some!"

This one hardly needs a recipe.

Servings: It depends on you!

Prep time: Maybe 30 minutes, max. Depends on how many you make, and how fast you can roll meatballs!

Ingredients:

extra-lean, ground turkey breast

1 package dry powdered Swedish meatball mix

All you do is prepare the meatballs according to the directions on the mix package. Substitute the turkey for beef, and substitute skim milk or reconstituted powdered nonfat buttermilk for the milk in the recipe. Brown the meatballs without oil on a nonstick griddle or in a nonstick pan. Use a spritz of spray oil if you want. To make them extra moist, simmer the meatballs in the sauce covered for ten minutes or so. Then remove the lid and let the sauce thicken up. Serve over brown rice or for a treat, splurge and serve the traditional way using yolkless noodles. (Yes, white pasta! I enjoy it, too, once in a while!) Try tossing a can of mushrooms into the sauce for some extra flavor! You will hardly miss the beef! If you want, substitute three-fourths of the beef with three-fourths of the extra-lean turkey and reduce that fat percentage by nearly 50 percent, while retaining some of the beef flavor! This works out to one part beef to three parts turkey.

Here are the numbers for four ounces of turkey balls (without the noodles):

Mel's "Svedish Meatballs, and then some!"		Traditional Meatballs with Beef	
Calories: 146		Calories: 313	
Protein: 30	(82%)	Protein: 29	(37%)
Carb: 4.5	(12%)	Carb: 4	(5%)
Fat: 1	**(6%)**	**Fat:** 20	**(58%)**

What to do with leftover turkey balls? Here are a couple of ideas: Toss them into some pasta sauce and instant spaghetti and meatballs! The pasta sauce will hide any of the Swedish sauce flavor.

Need lunch on the run? No problem. Got three or four meatballs left over? Put a few slices of nonfat mozzarella cheese (I prefer soy cheese because it melts!) on one side of the inside of a whole-wheat pita bread (cut the top of the bread off). Spoon in some pasta sauce. Cut your meatballs in half and stuff them in the pita pocket. Spoon more sauce over the meatballs. Sprinkle on some red pepper flakes if you want. Put it on a plate and nuke it for a minute or so. Instant meatball sandwich on the run. This one is really great.

Here's another idea: Cut the meatballs in half and use them to stuff zucchini boats (blanch the zucchini first, then finish off in the microwave or in the oven), or chop up the meatballs and use them to stuff a green pepper! Have a few leftover balls but no Svedish sauce? Heat the balls up in a can of low-fat cream of mushroom soup, or mix up a package of instant (powdered) mushroom gravy or turkey gravy. One more idea for you. "Nuke" the balls in the microwave, crumble them up, and use to stuff a soft taco or better yet, make a taco salad with some brown rice and the chopped up meatballs. Top with some salsa and nonfat cheese, and of course nonfat sour cream. See what you can do with a little old meatball?

Mel's "Give Me Griddled Cheese" Sandwich

Serves: 1 (makes two sandwiches)
Prep time: 15–20 minutes max!

Pull out that new nonstick griddle and have a burst of creative genius. Do whatever you want with this one. Do you love ooey, gooey, stringy melted cheese that tastes like real cheese? Make mine and you won't have a cheese craving for several days—no skimping here. Of course, you could lapse back into the diet mentality and use real, fat-laden cheese. To get the same calorie and fat count as mine, you wouldn't even be able to find the cheese! Why bother! Life is too short to be deprived of what you love.

Here we go!

4 slices (1 oz. each) of French bread

6–8 button mushrooms, sliced

3–4 good slices of a large, sweet white onion. We in the Northwest are proud of our Walla Walla Sweets! Nothing better!

½ of a large green pepper, cut into about one-half-inch-thick slices

2 oz. mozzarella-flavor soy cheese (nonfat. Check the labels.)

½ oz. of lower-fat regular cheddar cheese (about 6 fat grams per serving) or regular soy cheese (3–4 grams of fat per serving and use 1 ounce)

basil, fresh or dried

fresh (or in the jar) finely chopped garlic

salt and pepper

Heat up the griddle (medium-low to medium—don't get it too hot!) and give a light spritz of cooking spray. Place the peppers and onions on the griddle, evenly distributed so everything is in one layer. You can separate the onion rings at any time, or let them do it themselves. Lightly grind some salt and pepper over the top of the veggies. Sprinkle on a little bit of dried basil or a bit more of finely chopped fresh basil. If the veggies start to brown before they are getting soft, turn down the heat, move everything to the center of the griddle and cover with a large lid. I do this anyway. It keeps the veggies moist in "sweat." While the veggies are cooking, pull out the bread. On what will be the inside, spread on as much crushed garlic as you like. Turn and stir-fry the veggies. Grate the cheese. Turn and stir-fry the veggies. Throw in the mushrooms. (Hey, nothing worse than burnt veggies!) Put the cheese on the "insides" of the bread slices. If you are lucky and don't have "holey bread," put the cheese on all four slices so the sandwich will hold together more easily.

If you do have "holey bread" just divide the cheese up between two of the slices. Maybe you will get lucky like me and two out of four won't be "holey bread." Sorry, today is Sunday. When the veggies are soft, but still firm, and the onions and everything have caramelized, remove the veggies from the heat. Evenly divide the pepper strips between two slices of bread, then top the peppers with the onions and mushrooms. Put the "lids" on. Reheat that griddle over medium low heat (wipe it off with a paper towel first) and lightly spritz with spray oil. Place the sandwiches on the griddle and lightly spritz the tops with the spray oil. Allow these masterpieces to slowly cook, toast and turn a beautiful golden brown. The slower cooking allows all that cheese time to melt. Check the bottoms frequently. When the bottoms are browned, gently flip the sandwiches over. Use your fingers or a second flipper to help hold everything together just to make sure you don't lose one bite of anything. Continue to cook until the second side is golden. Remove to a plate, grab some paper towels (maybe a bib if you went overboard with the veggies) and indulge! You will know you have had lunch after this one. In fact, you may never want fat-laden, plain, old everyday cheese sandwiches again. For added variety, try some sourdough or whole-wheat French bread, or any of those gourmet breads out there, as long as they are very low in fat (I mean one gram of fat or less per serving). Experiment with different veggies. Try adding in some sprouts, red bell peppers, zucchini, eggplant, whatever is in season that will stay on a sandwich when cooked! You can even splurge and top the veggies before cooking with some sundried tomato (not packed in oil).

Here are the numbers:

Mel's "Give Me Griddled Cheese" Sandwich			Traditional Grilled Cheese Sandwich		
Calories:	450		Calories:	344	
Protein:	20	(21%)	Protein:	10	(12%)
Carb:	65	(69%)	Carb:	28	(37%)
Fat:	**5**	**(10%)**	**Fat:**	**19**	**(51%)**

Mel's "For The Love Of Stuffed Green Peppers"

Stuffed green peppers are one of those things either people love or hate. I love them, but I hate all of the fat in the traditional version. As summer draws to an end, and I feel that first bit of autumn crisp in the morning air, my thoughts turn to garden everything. My favorite fall meal is stuffed green peppers, corn on the cob, rice and a green salad with garden-fresh veggies. While growing up, Mom always fixed green peppers on Mondays (replacing Monday meatloaf for that season). Hers were the best, in my mind. She never put rice in hers, but even before I changed my lifestyle, and when I ate red meat, I still liked a bit of rice thrown into mine. This time, I didn't skimp on the meat so the fat content is somewhat up there, but when you calculate in the rest of the meal, and watch the fat for the rest of the day, you can easily still achieve 10 percent of calories or less for the entire day. Remember, it's not so much what you do at one meal but the totals over time that counts when it comes to fat. So eat what you love, and love what you eat!

Serving size: one large pepper
Number of servings: 1
Prep time: 5–10 minutes
Baking time: 30 minutes or less
Ingredients:
1 large green pepper, topped and seeded. (Save the top, toss the stem, chop up the flesh and set aside.)
4 oz. ground turkey (Look for the prepackaged kind that's low in fat, or have the butcher grind up some turkey (breast only), otherwise, you may end up with dark meat and lots more fat than you had planned on.)
¼ cup cooked short-grain brown rice (Something else to use that ¼ cup leftover for!)
3 slices of fresh sweet white onion, chopped
1 teaspoon or whatever of fresh or chopped garlic from a jar
1 teaspoon bread crumbs
salt and pepper

Stick the green pepper in a microwave-safe and oven-safe dish, add just a splash of water, cover with plastic wrap and "nuke" on high for one to one and one-half minutes, just until tender crisp. One reason people hate stuffed peppers is because they are overcooked. I don't like them that way either. Uncover the pepper and set aside. Heat a small nonstick pan over medium heat. Spritz with spray oil. Add the chopped onion, chopped pepper and garlic with a few grindings of salt and cook until the veggies are tender crisp, about five minutes. Crumble in the turkey meat, add fresh ground pepper to taste, and cook and stir just till the meat is no longer pink. Don't overcook it, and don't brown it. Remove from the heat and toss in the one-fourth cup of brown rice and mix well. Fill the pepper with meat mixture, pressing it into all of the nooks and crannies. Sprinkle the top with the bread crumbs and a spritz of spray oil. Put a tablespoon or so of water in the bottom of the dish. Place in a 350 degree oven just till hot and the bread crumbs start to turn golden brown,

20–30 minutes. Remove to a plate and enjoy! If you like, you can pour on tomato sauce before baking. Try putting some finely sliced mushrooms in the pan when the meat goes in. Do what you want. Do it the way you like it! You won't miss the beef at all!

Here are the numbers:

Mel's "For The Love of Stuffed Green Peppers"			Traditional Version		
Calories:	234		Calories:	361	
Protein:	22	(43%)	Protein:	21	(27%)
Carb:	15	(30%)	Carb:	7	(9%)
Fat:	**7**	**(27%)**	**Fat:**	**25**	**(64%)**

OK. So this meal was an afterthought. You already splurged with some fat for the day. No problem. Cut that fat in half again by substituting another one-fourth cup of brown rice for two ounces of the turkey meat. Maybe add some extra onion to the pan and a sprinkle of nonfat Parmesan on the top for added flavor. See, it's all about adapting what you like to meet what your body needs, without feeling deprived or hungry. That's BodyLogic!

Short on time? Sick of leftover Sunshine Meatloaf? Crumble up one serving slice of cold meatloaf and cram it inside of a raw green pepper. Stick it in a microwave safe dish with just a splash of water in the bottom. Cover with plastic wrap and nuke on high for five to six minutes. Dinner! You can't fix a green salad and "nuke" some veggies in that length of time!

Jan's "Salad Merger"

Serves: 4
Serving size: 1½ cups
Prep time: 5–20 minutes
Standing time: 30 minutes
Ingredients:

2 cups cooked (no-fat added, no-skin) cubed turkey breast
4 cups shell macaroni, cooked without fat, drained and cooled
1 cup broccoli, cooked without fat to tender crisp stage, cut into ½-inch pieces
1 cup raw sliced celery
4 Tbsp. Mel's Caesar Dressing (regular, not creamy)
½ packet aspartame if desired
½ tsp. sesame seeds

Cook the pasta and set aside to drain and cool. "Nuke" the broccoli at the same time and set aside to cool. In a large bowl, combine the turkey, broccoli and celery. Toss with the dressing mixed with aspartame if desired. Let stand thirty minutes. Sprinkle with toasted sesame seeds before serving.

Here are the numbers:

Jan's "Salad Merger" 1½-cup serving			Traditional Marinated Turkey Salad: ½-cup serving		
Calories:	258		Calories:	200	
Protein:	21	(36%)	Protein:	20	(46%)
Carb:	35	(61%)	Carb:	3	(8%)
Fat:	**1**	**(3%)**	**Fat:**	**10**	**(46%)**

Now we call that one a winner! For added variety, substitute brown rice for the pasta. Don't want pasta? That's fine, too. Jan's version will still have much less fat than the original.

Jan's "Sea Breeze" Salad

Serves: 8

Prep time: 30 minutes

Chill time: Whatever you like

Ingredients:

1 7-oz. package shell macaroni, cooked and drained

8 ounces of canned water-pack tuna

1 medium tomato, sliced

1 medium cucumber, sliced

1¼ cup diced, green pepper

¼ cup red onion slices (raw), separated into rings

1 tsp. salt

½ cup fat-free Italian dressing or Mel's Caesar Dressing

Cook the pasta according to package directions, without added fat, rinse and drain, set aside to cool. In the meantime, cut up the veggies. In a large bowl, mix the pasta, tuna, cucumber, green pepper, salt and dressing. Toss well to coat. Top with the onion rings and chill for as long as desired.

This one is really great on a hot summer's day for a terrific, light lunch or supper. It's also one of the best examples we have that show how simple it is to make just a few substitutions to achieve incredible outcomes. In this one, we cut the fat used in cooking the pasta. We substituted water-pack tuna for the regular tuna packed in oil. Finally, we substituted fat-free dressing for regular dressing. Tastes just about the same, but your body will love you for it!

Here are the numbers:

Jan's "Sea Breeze" Salad			Traditional Version		
Calories:	210		Calories:	366	
Protein:	12	(25%)	Protein:	12	(14%)
Carb:	35	(75%)	Carb:	37	(46%)
Fat:	**0**	**(0%)**	**Fat:**	**16**	**(40%)**

Mel's "The Cat's Meow Taco Salad"

Serves: 1

You want some dramatic numbers? I'll give you some. Summer always spurs on main-meal salad cravings for dinner. They are fast and filling, and usually loaded with fat. You know the typical ones: grilled chicken Caesar, oriental chicken, and everyone's favorite, taco salad! I'm no different than the rest of you. I love taco salad, even chicken fajita salad! How did this one get its name? I have a very funny Siamese cat named Sampson. One day several years ago, I made a pot of chili with beef and beans that was so hot, I could not eat it. When I turned my back, Sam got up on the counter (that *is* a no-no in my house!) and started licking the chili spoon! The cat went ape over the stuff. Ever since, he goes crazy whenever he smells anything that resembles the smell of chili. While creating this salad, once again Sam went nuts. I happily gave him some of the "meat" and he lapped it up and begged for more. Yup, I faked out the cat. I would bet money you will fake out your family as well with this one! Here's my version of the traditional beef taco salad. Eat to your heart's content!

Ingredients:

1 cup frozen meatless burger crumbles
1–2 Tbsp. powdered taco seasoning mix
½ cup chilled, leftover brown rice
sautéed onions (no fat added) as desired
lots of lettuce and tomato
1 ounce grated fat-free soy cheese
1 Tbsp. fat-free sour cream
as much salsa as you want
about 10 baked tortilla chips

In a preheated medium sauté pan, toss in one cup frozen meatless burger crumbles. You might luck out and find poultry, pork or beef flavors in the freezer section at the health food store or in the natural food section of your favorite market. Sprinkle in one or two tablespoons of powdered taco seasoning (I prefer the lower salt kind) and mix well. The more you add, the more you will believe it's the real McCoy!

Cook and stir until the "burger" starts to look like the real thing. It doesn't take long at all, maybe three minutes. When it's almost done, throw in one-half cup chilled leftover brown rice (separate it with your fingers like you would hamburger), separate the grains and stir occasionally until all is hot and smells wonderful. If it appears dry, sprinkle a tiny amount of water over and stir that in, maybe a couple of teaspoons. If you add too much water your mixture will resemble mush instead of beef! If you want, you can start the whole thing off with some sautéed onions.

While the "meat" is cooking, put some nice green and or red leaf lettuce in a large bowl. Cut up some chunks of tomato and throw that on top. Have some fun and place about ten bite-size baked low-fat (1 fat gram per serving) corn tortilla chips nicely around the sides. Make it look pretty! Save a chip or two for garnish. Grate up one ounce of nonfat cheese and set that aside. Throw the hot "meat" onto the top of the salad and sprinkle with the cheese. Top with as much salsa as you like.

I found a wonderful black bean and corn salsa—so nutritious, and fat free! Garnish with a tablespoon or two of nonfat sour cream and stand that last chip or two in the sour cream. ¡OLÉ! For added variety, replace one-half cup of the rice with one-half cup of canned black beans or pinto beans. Protein and fiber overload! If you prepare this for the family, kick them out of the kitchen while you are cooking. If they question the contents, just say you decided to stretch the meat budget and throw in some Mexican rice. They won't need to know what a stretch it is. After they beg for this salad several times, you can fess up if you want.

Now let's look at the numbers:

Mel's "Cat's Meow" Taco Salad			Original Version with Beef		
Serving size: 768 grams			Serving size: 760 grams		
Calories:	421		Calories:	1250	
Protein:	31	(35%)	Protein:	69	(21%)
Carb:	50	(57%)	Carb:	67	(21%)
Fat:	**4**	**(8%)**	**Fat:**	**78**	**(58%)**

You could eat nearly three times as much of mine (if you could hold it all) for the same number of calories as the original and still end up with about a fifth of the calories from fat. Is that totally amazing or what? Mine will fill you up. Brown rice is high octane fuel! Oh how your arteries will love you!

Mel's "Cat's Meow" Soft Tacos

Serves: 1

Use the same filling as for the salad above. Instead of the tortilla chips, use one fat-free corn or flour tortilla. This will add 50 calories, 1 protein gram and 12 carbo grams to the above numbers. Warm the tortilla in a dry, hot skillet for thirty seconds or so on each side.

Remove the tortilla to a plate and put the filling on the inside, top with the grated cheese and sour cream, and roll up the sloppy mess burrito style, leaving the top open. Put some lettuce in there if you want. Find your bib and dive in, using salsa freely, bite after glorious bite!

Get really adventurous and heat up a can of fat-free vegetarian refried beans and melt some nonfat jack cheese over the top. Yum! Add about 100 calories for a whole cup of beans and 30 calories or so for the cheese. Look on the can of beans for protein and carb numbers.

Mel's "Cat's Meow" Tostadas

Serves: 1

You got the picture. Same filling. This time, lightly spray the tortilla with some spray oil and stick it under the broiler for a short time until it becomes crisp and brown. Put it on a plate. Throw on the filling. Top with cheese, lettuce, tomato, sour cream and salsa. Same numbers as the tacos.

Mel's "Cat's Meow" Enchiladas

Serves: 1

Use a nonfat or low-fat corn tortilla, unheated. Put the "meat" filling (from previous recipes) in the center and wrap up all four sides, burrito style. Place seam side down in a baking dish lightly coated with spray oil. Pour over as much fat-free canned enchilada sauce as you like. Bake at 350 for thirty minutes or so, or until hot. Remove to an oven-safe plate. (Don't forget every last drop of the sauce!) Sprinkle grated nonfat cheese over the top and stick the enchilada back under the broiler just until the cheese is nearly melted. The heat from the enchilada will melt it the rest of the way by the time you eat. If you melt it the entire way under the broiler, the cheese may cool to a hardened mess. This generally does not happen with soy cheese. In fact, I have yet to find anything but soy cheese that melts worth a toot! So pull it out of the oven and top with salsa and sour cream as you like. You can sprinkle with some chopped jalapenos or green onions. Heck, go all out and sprinkle with a bit more cheese! Serve with some vegetarian refried beans (fat-free) with more cheese melted over the top of the beans if you are really in a cheese mode!

Mel's "Cat's Meow" Burritos...OK. Enough already! Nachos? I'm sure you get the idea by now. The opportunities are endless.

Mexican food is probably one of the easiest ethnic cuisines to adapt to low-fat, high-complex carbohydrate eating. Don't like the fake beef? Use fat-free refries or canned black or pinto beans and some brown rice for the filling, sprinkled with some of the taco seasoning. Use burrito seasoning. Try fajita seasoning. Do whatever you want. This is *your* food!

Had your fill of Mexican? What about Indian food? I told you I love ethnic food. It is high in flavor and low in fat. This curry will "kill" you.

Use this basic curry sauce, then add chicken, potatoes and peas, garbanzo's, shrimp, a bit of beef, eggplant, or whatever! I like my food very spicy. Adjust the cayenne pepper to your liking. Remember, you can always add more, but you can't take it away. If you get too crazy, add more tomato to the dish and/or extra plain yogurt to the finished product to cut the heat. Trust me, I've been there, done that. About had to call the fire department to put out the flame in my mouth! I'll give you the numbers for the chicken and shrimp versions. You can come up with numbers for whatever you like.

Mel's "Call-The-Fire-Department Curried Anything!"

Serves: 2

Prep time: 3 minutes

Cooking time: 5–10 minutes

Ingredients:

½ cup diced white onion (the sweeter the better!)

fresh, crushed garlic—as much as you want

Madras Curry Powder (not the cheap stuff *pleeze*!) 1–3 Tbsp. It's your call!

cayenne pepper to taste. Mel uses a good ½ tsp. but that's pure firewater. Again, your call.

½ can 98% fat-free chicken broth

6 oz. frozen, boiled shrimp or 6 oz. fresh chicken breast cut into cubes

cornstarch

water

salt to taste

plain, nonfat yogurt for garnish if desired

¾ cup cooked, short-grain or brown basmati rice

Heat a nonstick fry pan over medium low heat. Throw in the onions, sprinkle with a bit of salt, cover and let the onions "sweat" just until they are soft. Stir in the curry powder and cayenne and cook for about a minute, to release the flavor of those wonderful spices. Pour in the chicken broth and stir well. Just as the broth begins to boil, toss in the shrimp or chicken. Give a stir. Mix up a solution of one tablespoon cornstarch to one tablespoon water. Watch the curry mixture carefully. Don't overcook the meat. When the meat is nearly done, stir the cornstarch mixture into the pan. Keep stirring till the sauce is smooth and to your desired thickness. If you let it get too thick, just remove from the heat, stir in some water, then return to the heat for just a moment to bring it back to temperature. Remove from the heat and pour the whole mess over a nice plateful of short-grain brown rice, brown basmati rice, or rice of your choice. Garnish with the nonfat yogurt if desired. If you got carried away with the cayenne, the yogurt will put out the fire!

Serve it up with a green salad, and some whole-wheat pita bread or homemade *naan* if desired. (Naan is a wonderful fat-free Indian flat bread. It's best fresh out of the oven.)

Do whatever you want to this recipe. Add whatever meat or veggies you like. Garbanzo beans and spinach are wonderful added to curry. A real yummy meatless curry is made with fresh-diced potatoes and fresh or frozen green peas. Throw in some mushrooms, or cauliflower. You can make curry out of just about anything and it is very satisfying in the winter.

Here are the numbers:

Mel's "Call The Fire Department" Curry Shrimp version:			Traditional Curry:	
Calories:	213		441	
Protein:	24	(44%)	22	(21%)
Carb:	28	(54%)	45	(44%)
Fat:	**1**	**(4%)**	**17**	**(35%)**
Chicken version:				
Calories:	272		425	
Protein:	28	(45%)	22	(21%)
Carb:	28	(45%)	42	(42%)
Fat:	**3**	**(10%)**	**17**	**(37%)**

Mel's Linguini With Clam Sauce

Serves: 1

It doesn't get any easier than this folks. Who needs to go out to an expensive Italian restaurant and consume all of that fat in the process? Save over half the money and half the fat!

Ingredients:

2 oz. (dry) pasta of your choice. Try spelt grain, brown rice or corn varieties for added nutrition and no wheat (for those of you with wheat allergies).

½ cup prepared low-fat pasta sauce with extra garlic

½ cup whole baby clams (fresh, frozen or canned)

fat-free Parmesan cheese

If using frozen clams, thaw them in warm water while you are preparing the pasta.

Prepare the pasta according to the package directions, without adding any fat. While that's cooking, fix your salad, garlic toast, veggies or whatever.

Drain the pasta. In the same pan that you cooked the pasta (I'm lazy; I admit it.), dump in the pasta sauce, clams and extra garlic. Heat over low heat just until it bubbles, is hot, and the clams look cooked. Don't overcook the clams. Plate up the pasta, pour on the clam sauce, sprinkle with the cheese and you have a first class, gourmet Italian meal. I like mine with fat-free Caesar salad and garlic toast!

Get creative. Instead of red sauce, take a few extra minutes and fix white sauce. In a small saucepan, combine one-half cup canned evaporated skim milk, butter flavoring as desired, fresh crushed garlic as desired, salt and pepper. In a glass or something, mix up about one tablespoon of cornstarch and one to one and one-half tablespoons of water. Stir that in to the milk mixture. Bring the mixture to a slow boil over medium heat, stirring constantly until desired thickness. Toss in the clams and continue to cook just until the clams are cooked/ heated. Remove from the heat. Stir in a tablespoon or so of fat-free Parmesan cheese if desired. Toss with pasta. Not into clams? Keep the cheese, omit the clams, and you have fettucini alfredo!

Here are the numbers:

Mel's Linguini With Clam Sauce:			Traditional Version:		
Calories:	374		Calories:	465	
Protein:	18	(20%)	Protein:	21	(18%)
Carb:	56	(66%)	Carb:	63	(56%)
Fat:	**6**	**(14%)**	**Fat:**	**13**	**(26%)**

Mel's Smacaroni and Cheese

Serves: 2 (I like leftovers!)

Ingredients:

1 cup evaporated skim milk

2 Tbsp. cornstarch mixed with 2 Tbsp. water

4 ounces of nonfat soy cheese, any flavor you like, grated

butter-flavoring to taste

2 cups macaroni, cooked according to package directions, no added fat.

salt and pepper to taste

Prepare the pasta if you have not done so already. In the same pan, combine all of the liquid stuff and bring to a boil over medium heat, stirring constantly until nearly thick. Stir in the cheese and cook just until the cheese is melted. Season to taste with salt and pepper. Place the pasta in a baking dish spritzed with spray oil. Pour the whole liquid mess over the pasta and stir well. Top with a few more gratings of cheese if you like a crusty cheesy top. Bake at 350 for about thirty minutes or until heated through.

Here's a twist. Use the basic white sauce with or without the cheese. Toss in some sautéed onions and green peppers, some thawed frozen green peas, some pimiento and a can of water-pack tuna. Substitute eggless wide noodles for the macaroni. Sprinkle the top with a bit of fat-free Parmesan cheese and some bread crumbs. Tuna casserole to die for! See how one recipe becomes the basis for another?

Here are the numbers:

Mel's Smacaroni and Cheese			Traditional Version		
Calories:	220		Calories:	512	
Protein:	10	(18%)	Protein:	19	(15%)
Carb:	38	(82%)	Carb:	47	(38%)
Fat:	**0**	**(0%)**	**Fat:**	**26**	**(47%)**

The Grand Finale! (Dessert)

WARNING: The title of this next recipe may be inappropriate for some family members! You will keep them for yourself anyway!

This one is for adults only, ladies! When I tasted this, I said "Oh, man! Who needs men when I can have these?" Why should you share even one? If you try no other recipe, try this one. I guarantee you will be a convert for life! So how did this one come about? I had a chocolate brownie attack. I admit it. It happens on occasion. I'm human, OK? So I'm thinking, what has the same texture as the real thing? Pancakes, almost, but must be moister, creamier, fudgier. Then I think, OK, I created the muffins, let's take it once step further, or two! How could I get the moist, rich creaminess of chocolate fudge into an essentially fat-free recipe? What else has that flavor and creaminess? Then it hit me—chocolate fudge pudding! This was the result, after missing about two innings of my baseball game (the team was losing anyway!):

Mel's "Beyond Belief, Mile-High, Orgasmicly Triple-Chocolate Iced Brownies"

Yield: 12 brownies

Prep time: 5 minutes barely!

Bake time: 25–30 minutes

Cooling time: I couldn't wait that long! (At least 30 minutes in the fridge if you have more self control than I do!)

Ingredients:

1½ cups 10-Grain Pancake Mix (Here she goes again!)

3 Tbsp. cocoa powder

4-6 packages of aspartame

¼ cup (½ of a 1.4 ounce package) fat-free, sugar-free, instant chocolate fudge pudding mix

1½ cups buttermilk, nonfat (made from instant if necessary)

4½ Tbsp. (or ¼ cup and ⅛ cup) of egg substitute, fat-free

1 teaspoon almond extract (If you don't like nuts, use vanilla!)

Icing:

The other half package of pudding mix

¾ cup skim milk

4 Tbsp. fat-free cream cheese (regular flavor)

Preheat oven to 350 degrees.

In a medium bowl, mix together the dry ingredients. Make a well in the center. Pour the wet ingredients in and mix with a spoon just until well blended. Pour into a 8 x 8 inch square pan sprayed with cooking spray or lined with parchment if you need to. Spread the batter evenly around the pan and throw it in the oven. Bake for about twenty-five to thirty minutes, just until a pick inserted in the center comes out clean and the top is springy. Don't overbake. Cool on a wire rack for about ten minutes then stick it in the fridge until thoroughly cool. While that cools—use restraint, ladies!

To make the icing

Place the cream cheese in a small bowl and stir it up for a few seconds, just until it kind of collapses and is really creamy, kind of the consistency of nonfat sour cream or mayo. In another bowl, place the three-fourth cup *cold* skim milk. Add the cream cheese to the milk and mix with a hand mixer or hand blender for a few seconds, just until the cream cheese is incorporated and everything is kind of foamy. Sprinkle the rest of the pudding mix over the milk mixture and continue to mix until very well blended, about two to three minutes. The frosting will set up in the bowl by the time it is mixed. You may need to mix by hand with a rubber spatula to finish it off. This should be very creamy. If it's not sweet enough, add some aspartame to it. Mine came out quite sweet without additional sweetener! Immediately stick the frosting in the fridge. When the brownies are cool, top with *all* of the frosting (don't forget to lick the spoon) and return the whole thing to the fridge until ready to eat. The frosting will stay pudding-like for the first twenty-four hours or so, it is a bit messy. Use a fork if you are not into the primitive pleasure of eating with your fingers. If you are like me, you won't make it past the cooling stage. I had to try it with lukewarm brownies and cold frosting that melted all over it. Yum! Give me death by chocolate, please!

Not rich enough for you? Think of it as cake, put it on a plate and top with some fat-free whipped topping and a sprinkle of cocoa powder. Still not enough chocolate for you? Try this. Put a squirt or two of chocolate syrup (light, of course) on the bottom of a plate. Quadruple chocolate fudge brownies. Try these variations and think you really have died and gone to heaven:

Serve with some puréed raspberries, fresh strawberries, fresh banana, just a tiny sprinkle of coconut, a very few slivers of almonds, a bit of flavored syrup (like what you put in an espresso or Italian soda, like cherry or raspberry or whatever), and for holidays, try a teaspoon or two of your favorite liquor under your brownie such as Irish Cream, Grand Marnier, almond, kahlua, crème de coconut, peppermint schnapps, crème de cacao—my, my, oh my. Another variation? Put the flavored syrup or liquor right into the batter before baking. Add some instant coffee granules or replace the almond extract with coffee extract. Heck, use both! Do whatever you want to. This is *your* guilt-free comfort food! Still not enough variation for you? Make any flavor brownie you want. Use banana or pistachio pudding mix instead. Use the chocolate brownie batter and use a different flavor pudding mix for the frosting. Put the syrup or liquor in the frosting (you may have to decrease the milk a bit if you add a liquid flavoring).

OK. One more then I'll stop (actually I can't stop!): My Rx for the-worst-attack-of-PMS-you-ever-had: Quintuple Chocolate Brownies! Do like the "cake," and serve it on top of a couple of scoops of fat-free, sugar-free, chocolate frozen yogurt.

Can't eat just one? You don't have to! Just remember balance. Nothing but high-quality food here.

We promised you would never diet again!

Be sure to store these in the fridge (uncovered so they set up), to retain their ooey, gooey, chewy texture and to keep the "icing" from melting! The longer they stay in the fridge, the better they get!

Here are the unbelievable numbers:

Mel's "Iced" Brownies			Traditional Iced Brownies		
Each brownie contains:					
Calories:	81		Calories:	350	
Protein:	6	(30%)	Protein:	4	(4%)
Carb:	13	(68%)	Carb:	50	(54%)
Fat:	**1**	**(2%)**	**Fat:**	**16**	**(42%)**

We Scream for Banana Cream!

(A joint effort, on a weekend, in our PJs, while writing this book!)

Serves: 6

4 large wonton wrappers
2 small boxes of fat-free, sugar-free banana pudding mix
3 small bananas
3 cups skim milk

Layer the wrappers over the bottom and sides of a glass pie plate. Give a spritz of spray oil between each layer. Bake at 350 just until golden. Allow to cool. Slice up the bananas in the bottom of the crust. Prepare the pudding mix for pie filling as it says on the package, using skim milk. Pour the pudding over the bananas and chill. Top with fat-free whipped topping if desired.

Here are the numbers!

The traditional version:			We Scream for Banana Cream		
Calories:	490		Calories:	133	
Protein:	9	(7%)	Protein:	6	(17%)
Carb:	66	(54%)	Carb:	28	(82%)
Fat:	**21**	**(39%)**	**Fat:**	**<1**	**(1%)**

Mel's Simple Decadence!

Serves: 1
Prep time: 2 minutes
Cooking time: None

No time to cook and you have dinner guests? Here is a ridiculously simple dessert that everyone will love!

Ingredients:

1 pear, fresh and ripe!
About 1 Tbsp. reduced-calorie chocolate syrup
About 2 Tbsp. fat-free nondairy whipped topping

Peel and halve the pear. Remove the core. Place the pear inside up in a pretty fruit or dessert dish. Drizzle the chocolate syrup over the pears, then put a large blob of the whipped topping on the top of everything. Sprinkle on some cocoa powder if you like for extra glamour!

The numbers? Just 122 calories, 30 grams of carbohydrates, no protein, no fat! Pure pleasure!

Mel's Doughnuts

Sit down and stop laughing. Use the basic brownie recipe! This really is all purpose quality food, isn't it! If you don't want chocolate doughnuts, use vanilla pudding or banana pudding. Experiment! Try the white chocolate flavor! So how do you get something from a batter into something with a hole? Easy. Look around in specialty kitchen stores, and you will find mini-bundt pans. They look kind of like muffin pans only they have the bundt shape with the tube-thing in the middle. Just yesterday, we ran across mini Jell-O ring molds, but for the $3.50 each, we say stick with the bundt molds! Spray the pan with a good shot of cooking spray. Pour the batter in about one-fourth full and give another quick squirt of spray on the tops, to give that same texture as a fried doughnut, and bake as usual. It probably won't take quite as long as the regular brownies. These obviously come out as a cake-type doughnut. If you like something sweet on your doughnuts, try brushing the tops with fruit-based sweetener as soon as they come out of the oven. You can splurge and give a light dusting of powdered sugar if you want. Or, keep a bowl of the brownie icing in the fridge and spread it on top each time you eat a doughnut.

Something else that's tasty is just to mix some aspartame into a bit of nonfat cream cheese. That gives a nice, sweet, creamy topping!

Using the brownie recipe, your numbers will be equivalent to two brownies for each donut, icing included. If you skip the icing, deduct about 30 calories. No fat in the icing.

Here's a challenge for you. You work on the "bread" type donut recipe. See if you can come up with something wonderful, and submit it to our newsletter. (See page 255 for information about how to reach us.)

We could go on forever with recipe examples. We hope we have given you ideas to adapt your own favorites to a healthier way of eating. The golden rule? Eat if you are hungry! Don't worry about eating too many calories as long as you are moving your body and listening to what it is telling you!

Part Two

Custom Body Detailing

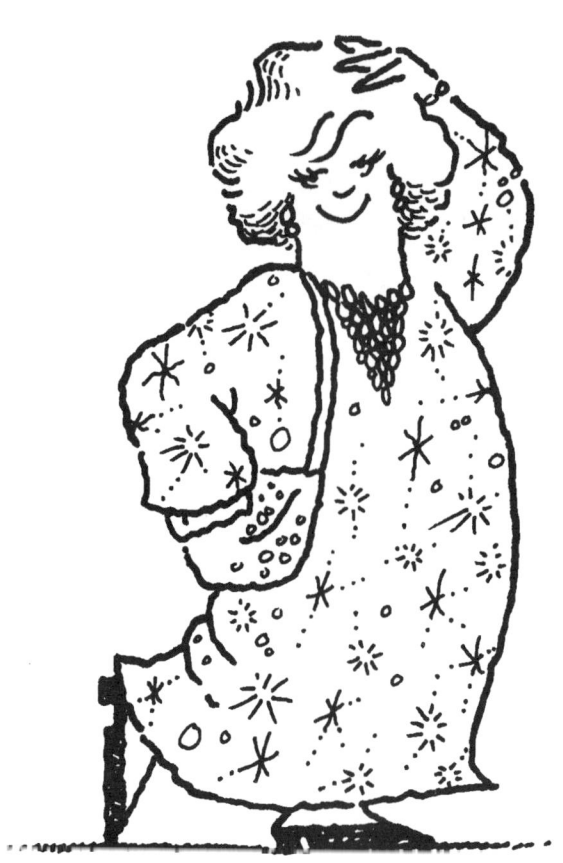

From Clunker to Classic

The Fine Art of Body Work

Let's face some cold, hard facts about having a fat body. We have explained in depth how the mind influences the body to change. Gaining control over the mind is the one most important step in changing your lifestyle. Let's move away from the topics of food, and into body image. You can't expect others to accept and respect you if you do not accept and respect yourself. The appearance of the exterior, and the words that come out of our mouths are what makes us fat people in the eyes of others. You must first like yourself, and this like of self must be reflected in how you look and how you act.

Previous mention has been made about the very real issue of fat discrimination in our society today. Overweight people are unfortunately often seen as unhealthy and/or dirty. One prime example is applying for a life insurance policy. How many overfat people are turned down entirely due to their weight, even though their doctor has given them a clean bill of health? We are often viewed as a "high risk." Have you ever been denied a seat on a charter plane tour because your weight would cause the weight limit of the aircraft to be exceeded? Have you ever been denied a place on a fishing boat tour because no life jacket would fit you? Have you ever felt you were turned down for a job, lost a job or failed to advance in your job because of your weight? Were you ever denied health insurance or charged an outrageous premium because you were considered high-risk? These are some very real issues, most of which we can change.

Unfortunately, some of us bring on these perceptions ourselves. Remember the saying, "You only get one chance to make a good first impression"? For overfat people, our first impressions often have to be better than those of our skinny counterparts if we are to get what we want. It seems we have to work twice as hard to prove ourselves in many situations. Consider how you view other fat people! We often judge each other with the same prejudiced attitude that skinny people judge us by. That is a real sad fact isn't it? The very people who need our support the most are the ones we are least likely to associate with! What's even worse is to make friends only with other fat people, often those people with the same kind of commitment to self care that we have. Yet another protective layer of armor! The first step in overcoming fat discrimination starts with each of us. As stated in another part of this book, if you change how you feel about yourself, your improved self-image will draw others to you. If you improve the appearance of the outside of your body (and we are not talking fat loss and muscle gain), it will change not only how others interact with you, but how you interact with others.

Whom would you be more drawn to:

1. A woman at the grocery store in curlers, too-tight sweat pants and sloppy shoes, or
2. A woman in a nicely fitting, clean dress with pantyhose, shoes in good repair, hair and makeup appropriate for the occasion?

Whom would you be more drawn to:

1. A male waitperson with greasy hair, body odor and a nose ring, with dirty jeans and untied shoelaces, or
2. A male waitperson with clean, twill trousers, a well-pressed sport shirt, neatly groomed hair and shoes in good repair?

What is the first thought that crosses your mind when you see a large woman walking down the street with no bra on, too-tight pants and a top that does not cover her belly? What is the first thought that crosses your mind when you see a large man walking down the street with his pants half-sliding off his backside and his belly hanging over his belt? Are these people ones you would want to chat with at a bus stop or in line at the grocery store? And even if you did choose to strike up a conversation with anyone, no matter what they looked like, how long would you keep your interest if their body odor nearly blew you over?

Try this experiment. Put on your grubbiest clothes, skip your shower and makeup, and go to a higher-class department store in search of a new piece of clothing to wear to work. How long will it take you to be approached by a clerk? Look at how busy the store is in comparison to your wait time. How friendly was the clerk? Did she talk to you like a person, engage you in conversation or did she rush through the encounter and push you into buying something you really did not like?

A week later, repeat the experiment, this time after careful washing and grooming, wearing clothing you would wear to a high-profile sales meeting. Pretend you just got off work or were on your lunch break. Were you treated any differently this time?

Now consider your attitude in your grubbies versus your better clothes. In which clothing were you more outgoing? More friendly? More personable? Which clothing made you feel better about yourself? Was your posture improved wearing the nicer clothes?

Granted, our skinny counterparts have just as many annoying and disgusting hygiene habits as we do. Not all fat people present this way in public, however, one rotten apple will spoil the whole barrel. In order to overcome the discrimination we face on a daily basis, and in order to achieve a successful lifestyle change, one of the easiest choices you can make is to improve how you look—not only to others, but to yourself.

We are going to take the liberty of talking to you candidly about some very personal topics, likely things your parents never taught you! OK, maybe they did, but you were too stubborn or too much in denial to really hear what they were saying!

Wash and wax

The first step needs to be into the shower! This means shampoo and condition the hair, wash every body part with soap or an appropriate cleanser. Pay special attention to places where skin meets skin, to areas that rarely see the light of day. (We know where those are, folks!) Are there any body parts that have not felt the soothing sensation of a shower spray in some time? Maybe never? Is there any part of a baby's lower anatomy that you would neglect during a bath or diaper change? Your body is no less important! Start from the top and work down, and don't forget the feet! If you have skin allergies, consult with your physician as to which products you should use. Shave what needs to be shaved. Ladies, this may mean your face. This is nothing derogatory. Hormones can get out of whack, resulting in excess body hair in places we would rather not see it!

You have learned to listen to your body to learn what fuel it needs. Now you must learn to differentiate the odors and appearance of each of your body parts. Know what is normal and what is not. If you notice an odor, likely others will too! If a good bath, shaving/trimming of body hair, deodorant and/or foot powder do not fix the problem, please talk with your physician. You may have an infection that may need to be treated. This should not be embarrassing. There is absolutely nothing a physician has not seen, heard or smelled before!

Bacteria breed in places that are warm and moist, places that do not get air and that do not stay dry. This results in obnoxious odors, skin rashes and infections. So step out of the shower, towel off with a clean dry towel in every place you can reach, and use a blow dryer in places you cannot. If you need to, pull apart skin folds and dry them well. Now pamper yourself with your favorite talc or just plain cornstarch. Babies find it soothing and refreshing, so do we. Flaky skin looks unhealthy. Flaky skin can result in small skin breaks that can cause infection. Everyone should follow their shower with a moisturizer appropriate for their skin type (both face and body). If you are prone to acne or skin breakouts, overly dry skin will only worsen the problem. An oil-free moisturizer will help reduce breakouts. Again, check with your physician if you have skin allergies.

Use an antiperspirant and deodorant under your arms and on the bottoms of your feet if your feet are prone to sweat and odor. Ladies, be cautious of feminine powders, sprays and other products. Often these cause more harm than good. These products may mask a serious problem or they may cause skin irritation. Worse yet, they may upset the natural pH balance of the area, resulting in more infections and skin problems. Odor problems emanating from private places are best managed by soap and water, as well as the trimming of excess body hair.

One last area not to be neglected is your mouth. As you change your foodstyle, you may temporarily experience some difficulties with breath odor. This will resolve in time as your body adjusts to its new fuel source, unless you are like your authors and are addicted to garlic and onions! Floss, and brush your teeth and tongue. Do this a minimum of twice a day, more often if needed. If you have a history of breath odor problems, or if these problems do not seem to resolve with these self-help measures, visit your dentist. You may need a more thorough cleaning, restorative care, or may have a gum disorder. Mouthwashes are a personal choice. Often times they only mask a potentially serious problem!

Roof care

One of the best investments you can make is one good trip to a quality hairstylist to learn which of the current styles best fits you and your lifestyle. You will want to keep it simple and easy to care for. Hair that requires more than fifteen minutes to fix likely will not be fixed on a regular basis! Make sure the style fits the shape of your face. A good cut can make all the difference in preventing "cave person" syndrome! Mother Nature may not have necessarily gone to hairstyling school. Whether you are female or male, take a good hard look at what nature gave you and then allow yourself the choice to cover that gray or enhance or even change your hair color. A little bit of sparkle really makes you shine!

You do not have to spend a lot of money to change and maintain your new look. Shop around. Learn what style is best and if you need to, go to a less costly salon and train your new hairstylist to give you the quality cut you deserve. Shop at beauty supply stores for quality products at lower costs. The hair tonic or conditioner that you find on sale at the grocery store may actually cause dandruff or other problems. Experiment and you will find quality products at reasonable prices. Also, keep in mind that many of us use much more shampoo, conditioner, mousses and gels than we actually need. A small amount of a quality product goes a long way. When you think the bottle of shampoo or conditioner is empty, put a bit of water in it and shake it well. You will be amazed at how many more days of use you will get out of those bottles. The same holds true for toothpaste, cosmetics, aftershave, deodorant and other personal care products—less is more!

A windshield with cracks and dings?

OK. Let's evaluate how well Mother Nature did with your facial features. You do not have to look like a movie star every time you leave the house. Blotchy, pale skin makes you look unhealthy. If you were blessed with perfect skin, rosy cheeks and long eyelashes, you should rejoice and go *au naturale!* But let's face it, few of us were born with those blessings. Even if you were, a bit of foundation or sunscreen is a must to protect you from the damaging effects of the sun and prevent premature aging of the skin. You have enough wrinkles on your body already. Why do you need any more? Not to mention what skin cancer can do to you! You do not have to spend a lot of money to give yourself what Mother Nature forgot. A bit of foundation, some blush, mascara and a bit of lip color will go a long way in making you feel better and look better. The goal is to enhance what nature gave you, not make yourself ready to look good in front of a camera! Men, this applies to you, too. More and more specialty stores are available to assist you in improving your appearance and the health of your skin. An occasional trim of the beard and mustache will improve your appearance 100 percent!

Undercoating!

Now that your skin and hair have received their daily dose of special attention, it's time to get ready to face the world! Let's move on and check out what is in the underwear drawer! You were probably taught to change your underwear every day! Our mothers always said cleanliness is next to godliness. They also said, "Never be caught in the hospital emergency room with dirty, ragged underwear!" We nurses know we could care less about the condition of someone's underwear, but *you* might care and *your* feelings are what's important! This is not just a hygiene issue! The condition of your underclothes is like a coat of primer on bare wood. Underclothes improve the look, feel and durability of outerwear. Besides, good underclothes also can give you lift and support that nature forgot or that you have lost over time. This applies to women as well as to men. We all have lots of wonderful options out there to help support what needs supporting, lift what needs lifting, and smooth out what needs smoothing! Quality undergarments will make even inexpensive clothing look like a million bucks.

Hey, clothing manufacturers, take note: you are sewing ladies undergarments and making pantyhose with the wrong side of the fabric on the outside! Ladies, if your slip rides up and your thighs sound like a freight train coming down the tracks when you walk, try putting those garments on inside out! The problem may not be a too small size! We promise you, if that's the problem, the slip will no longer go north and the hose will be less likely to move east and west! If the hose go south, they *are* the wrong size. If your thighs turn to raw meat when you wear pantyhose, it is due to the friction of chubby thighs rubbing together. Whether you choose to call them bloomers, pettipants, split slips, pant slips or pant liners, you know what they are. Experiment with wearing them either under your hose or over your hose. They will help prevent skin breakdown and they may also extend the life of those expensive hose. Keep shopping for hose until you find the proper fit. Keep the packages so you know what you have tried. There are hose on the market made for 5'10" 450-pound women. Your size is available! All you have to do is find it! Wash your hose before you wear them. This adds elasticity and prevents runs. Hand wash your hose and bloomers in gentle detergent after each wearing.

Gentlemen, let's not leave you out of the picture. Get socks that fit at your specialty departments or stores. Loose socks look sloppy. Nothing looks worse than a man's hairy leg exposed above the sock and below the pant leg. You may not see it, but we do!

Men and women, take note. Good hosiery does more than protect your feet from rubbing against your shoes. Tight socks impair circulation in your feet and can result in some very dangerous foot disorders and infections. This is extremely important in diabetics, if you want to keep your legs. Choosing fabrics that wick away moisture reduces foot odors!

While we are on the subject of underwear, nothing looks more tacky, for either males or females, than to see undergarments through your clothes. This can be a direct view, or it can be lines and wrinkles created from garments that do not fit correctly, are worn out or are poorly made for the clothing you put over them. Cover what needs to be covered, and select underwear appropriate for outerwear. Wear full briefs under slacks to avoid underwear lines!

A new coat of paint for your vehicle

Now that we have given you several very good reasons to clean out your underwear drawer, let's get you dressed and go shopping!

Make sure your clothes are clean and in a state of good repair. Ditch the safety pins and replace hooks, snaps and buttons. Repair zippers and close up the seams. You don't have to be able to sew or spend a lot of money to make many of these repairs. Go to a large fabric store and ask for help with choosing the right products. If you are prone to underarm perspiration, purchase an inexpensive pair of "dress" shields. These can be attached in a variety of ways. Again, ask for help. Clothing is too expensive to allow a bit of embarrassment to get in the way.

Now get dressed, check yourself in the mirror, put on a smile and head out to learn how to decorate your beautiful body. Visit a quality store that carries your size and style. You deserve to have at least one nice set of clothes. Consult with the salesperson if you need to regarding the style, size and color best suited to your body type, skin and hair color, and most of all, tastes. Try on the clothes. If you plan to make a purchase, do not hesitate to ask for any alterations needed. Have the salesperson look at you in your new duds to make sure the clothes fit you properly. Better yet, make this an extra fun day. Take a trusted friend with you to keep you on track and give you honest feedback about any items you plan to purchase.

Make sure you choose easy-care fabrics that breathe and tend not to wrinkle. Make sure the seams are well constructed. Most of all, make sure you really like what you plan to purchase. It won't do any good for your wallet or your self-confidence to have new clothes sitting in the closet and not adorning your body. Finally, plan a special event for your new attire. It could be as simple as having a few friends over for a healthy gourmet meal.

The sky is your limit. You can choose to be put down, or you can choose to go after what you want! A healthy, attractive appearance starts on the inside. You can be fat and good looking! Go for it!

Your positive self statement for today: Every day in every way, I get better and better!

Headlights

In this chapter we will discuss the proper fitting and caring for a bra, in addition to the health of the breast. Jan tried to come up with various titles for this chapter such as "Over The Shoulder Boulder Holder"; "Double Barrel Sling Shot"; "Point 'Em Up And Move Em Out"; The Strap That Binds"; "Look 30 Pounds Lighter, Buy a Bra That Fits" and "Get It Off Your Chest." No matter what the title, the following information will keep what's up front pointing in the right direction!

Proper fit of a bra is essential for the health of the breast. The breast comes in all shapes, sizes and densities. There basically are two kinds of bras: good ones and bad ones. There are many different styles; underwire and soft cup are the main ones, stretch straps, demi-bras, sport bras and nursing/maternity bras. Bra sizes can range from 32 to 56 and "A" cups to "I" cups. These sizes are available without having to purchase expensive specialty bras.

There are different bras for different body styles. If a woman is long-waisted, an underwire bra can be the best for her, especially if she is full-breasted. This style of bra lifts the breast from underneath thus taking the weight and stress off the shoulders and upper back. The wire does the work, not her body. But remember, this bra is not for every woman.

Soft-cup bras come in many different styles. Some have soft, pillowy support under the breast that attempts to push the breast up from the bottom to give it uplift. Others have support that circles the breast starting from the top of the cup and going around, thus lifting the breast from the top of the bra.

Stretch-strap bras can be good or bad. The drawback of them is that the stretchy strap allows for the breast to bounce with each step taken, thus allowing for breast tear-down. If a women is smaller-breasted, yet fuller-banded around, this can be a good bra. The woman with sloping shoulders quite often finds this style of bra good, but remember this type of strap can also dig deeply into the shoulder, even down to the shoulder blade.

Demi-bras or shelf bras are not readily available in the fuller sizes. This style of bra (in our opinion) is designed for the evening dress. We do not feel it is supportive enough for daily wear, and under certain fabrics can allow an improper sighting. Bosoms in this type of bra do not belong in the work place.

A full-breasted woman (size DD to I) very seldom will be "lifted and separated" such as the commercials suggest. There is too much breast. And ladies, look at the women in those commercials; they are "A", "B", or "C" sized breast. If an "I" breast were to be separated, the bosom would be pointing east and west instead of due north!

If you do not know what size bra you really need, find a specialty shop that will help you. Make sure your clerk really knows what she is doing. Find someone near your own age if possible. This way you will feel more comfortable and she will understand your needs. There are some specialty bras out there where the clerk needs to put the bra on you, thus touching your breasts. This is also your "Driver Education" class where you will learn how to put the bra on correctly. Try to remember the size of bra you were last wearing. This can help your clerk a lot.

Some clerks are so good they can pretty well size you up without measuring. They may ask you several questions and then hand you a starting bra. Remember all bras fit differently and will size out differently. Trust your clerk. She just might know what she is talking about!

Unfortunately, good bras do cost money. Specialty bras can run $50 to $70, while commercial bras can run $25 to $35. There are fifty different pieces that go into making a bra. Try to build up a bra wardrobe. Yes, get all the colors that are available. Always white and black. Depending on the beige color, you will also want this color in your wardrobe. If the beige is very yellow, it will show through your white tops. Try to have at least seven bras, one for each day of the week. This way you have a clean bra for each day of the week. Do you not change your panties daily? Then why not change your bra daily? If you don't think your bra is dirty after one wearing, wear a bra color the opposite of your skin tones and look how dirty it really is. That will prompt you for a daily changing! Body oils help wear out a bra, too. This is why a bra needs to be washed after each wearing. The life of one bra is three months. Yes! It is dead after three months. It is stained and droopy. If you cannot afford a clean bra for each day of the week, hand wash your bras daily, but do get them into the washing machine at least once a week for a good scrubbing. Be sure to fasten the hooks and eyes (especially with the underwire bras) so they don't go all over the machine getting stretched and twisted out of shape.

NEVER, NEVER, NEVER dry your bras in the dryer. Heat and elastic do not go together! This is like taking a $50 bill and throwing it out the car window going 70 mph—you will never get it back.

When trying on a new bra, look for bubble over the top of the cup, as well as armpit pillow. Should either of these situations occur, then the bra cup is too small for you. The armpit pillow is not body fat, but actual breast tissue and needs to be in the cup of the bra. If in your last bra you had the pillowy tissue hang over, it will take eight to twelve weeks for the crease to go away, once a new bra fits correctly. Support the breast. Some women have a lot of tissue under the armpit. Once this tissue is in the bra cup where it belongs, you may actually have a bust line! Another sign of a bra not fitting correctly is the bra riding up the back. The band needs to be smaller, but the cup may also need to be increased, sometimes one cup size, sometimes several cup sizes. Consult your bra-fitting expert.

Jan owns and operates a Plus-size lingerie and casual clothing store, Absolute Woman, in Portland for ladies 200 to 500 pounds. She has expertise in properly fitting the everyday bras and nursing bras. Jan notes that approximately 85 percent of the women who visit her store for the first time are wearing the wrong size bra, and many report that they have never undergone a professional fitting.

Various studies have been done during the last twenty-five years that indicate that 70–80 percent of women are wearing the wrong size bra. That is a huge percentage. Don't be a part of the statistic.

When you put a bra on, whether you reach around and hook it, or hook it in front and slide it around your body, there are a few tricks to getting the breast in the cup the correct way. Lean over slightly. Take your right hand and reach into the left bra cup to underneath the arm pit. Gently pull this breast tissue into the cup of the bra. Repeat on the other side. If you are fuller breasted, more than a "DD" never, never shake your breasts in any shape or form. (No pun intended.) This will allow the breast tissue to tear and before long your breast will reach your navel (or lower)!

Once your bra is on, regardless if it is 5:00 A.M. or noon, and you take it off twelve to eighteen hours later, you should never have to adjust yourself or the bra at all. Your bra should fit you so nicely that you forget you have it on. Yes! It is possible!

Some ladies experience a yeast-like infection under the breast, commonly caused by wearing a soiled bra. This is especially common in warmer weather. In your local drug store there are antibacterial soaps available. Read the instructions carefully and rinse very well. As a rule, the yeast-like infection usually clears up in three to five days. See your doctor before self-treating any new condition.

Sport bras

One of the most important purchases you can make when starting your new lifestyle is a well-fitting sports bra. All of the same rules apply. Make sure it fits, and that it is comfortable and provides excellent support. Any good bra also can be worn as a sports bra. The idea of this type of bra is to keep the bosom in the least amount of movement while being active. The two kinds of bras we have seen are the slip over the head type and the ones with real cups with hooks and eyes in the back. Either type is fine; but, these usually top out in a "DD" cup and that is it. So you ask what is the fuller-breasted woman to do? Here is where you get a little creative. Find a good everyday bra with great support. Once you have the bra on in the dressing room, jog or jump around. Try to simulate whatever type of activity you will be doing to test the bra for support. If this type of bra is not possible to find, then look in the local drug store for a three-inch-wide elastic bandage and bind you bosom to your body. Make sure you do not wrap yourself too tightly or you could cut off circulation to the tissues and impair breathing. Nothing draws more attention to a large or small woman's body than her boobs flapping in the wind as she moves. Trust us, men do notice, and not necessarily in a positive manner! One method or another will keep your bosom from bouncing all over the place and tearing down the breast tissue, especially as your activity tolerance increases. *Never* do physical activity without some type of support for your bosom. Torn tissue results in sagging breasts, and most of us have enough stuff sagging already! Jiggling breasts cause discomfort, and lack of support can result in neck and upper back pain. Try to find a bra of breathable fabric. This will help to prevent skin irritations, not to mention reduce odor. Remember, we do not want nipple, belly button, nipple.

Did you hear the joke: "What size of bra is worn in a nursing home? 36-long!"

Nursing bras

When pregnancy occurs a woman needs to pay special attention to her bosom. No two women's pregnancies or bosoms will do the same things; in fact, even your own two or three pregnancies will be different. Do not compare yourself to your mother, sister, cousin or aunt. No two bodies are the same. Some women's breasts start out a "B" cup and will increase to an "H." After breast feeding is finished, some bosoms will go back to the pre-pregnancy size. Others will not.

Regardless, as your breasts swell with pregnancy, remember to always have a properly fitting bra. Some women will increase their bra size all at once, while others will do so more gradually.

Protect your breasts during this very important and wonderful time. Remember this will be the baby's breakfast table. Droopy breasts can be prevented with a properly fitting bra.

About one month before your baby is due, you will want to select your nursing bras. There should be just a small amount of room left in the cup for a nursing pad. There are washable pads available as well as disposable varieties.

Think of a brand-new, clean baby and keep your breast clean and healthy. Have at least two nursing bras as one will always be in the wash.

Cancer prevention

As we are all aware, the American Cancer Society encourages us to do a monthly breast exam just after our periods. If you have reached menopause and no longer have periods, schedule your self-exam for the same date each month. Ask your physician or other health care practitioner to teach you how to correctly do an exam. Ask your OB/GYN to feel what you do in your breasts so you will know in your own breast what is normal. Breast exams are simple—cancer is not!

Ladies, if you do not know how to do a breast self-exam, then you are long overdue for a checkup! Make an appointment to see your doctor or health care provider *today*. We cannot stress this enough. Did you know the majority of breast cancers are discovered by women themselves, during their monthly exams? These cancers are caught early, often long before they are noticeable on mammography. Early detection means greater chances for a cure. This is nothing to take lightly. Once you master self-examination, teach it to your daughters. The gift of life did not stop the day they were born.

You may have heard reports recently that underwire bras can cause breast cancer. It may not be the bra itself, but the fit that may be a contributing factor. The jury is still out on this one. We have not personally seen any studies regarding the relationship between soft cup bras and breast cancer. Common sense tells us that a poorly fitting bra certainly can cause boils, cysts and other types of skin infections and irritations. For what it's worth, an ounce of prevention is worth a pound of cure. Take any steps you can to prevent such disorders, and protect your neck, back and shoulders in the process. Make sure your bra fits you perfectly.

One final note

The topic of "Headlights" is not for women only! Gentlemen, this is a very delicate subject to address, but you, too, should be examining your breasts on a monthly schedule. Yes, men have been know to die from breast cancer. Another thing to consider is wearing a bra. It will take a special sales clerk to help you, but let her know your concern and the incidence of this disease in men is on the rise. Call ahead and be sure to give her your name in full at the beginning of the call. Unfortunately, there are a lot of prank callers and cross-dressers calling for bras all the time, so the clerk's guard will be up. If you have difficulty finding a clerk who will help you, a note from your physician should validate your need. Be pleasant and know what you are talking about. You will get the clerk's respect and then you can proceed with explaining your concerns and needs.

Packing the Essentials

Some Final Words

You have spent a long time and expended a lot of energy getting ready to embark on your new life's journey. The road will be full of twists and turns, ups and downs, with a few potholes thrown in just to keep things interesting. Hopefully, you won't run into many major construction delays or severe storms along the way. You are ready! You have prepared your vehicle inside and out. You have your maps, your route determined and many exciting side trips planned. So, you may think there is only one thing left to do. Get packed, right? Wrong! You have already done that! You have filled your trunk with some very precious cargo. Lock it up. Don't ever lose it. This cargo cannot be taken from you unless you are careless with it. Have the most wonderful adventure of your life!

Don't ever let fear get in the way of what you really want in life. The process happens so slowly, so naturally, that you will adapt to your new body and lifestyle without even knowing it. It's kind of like setting the cruise control along with the auto pilot. One day, you will be amazed at how far you have traveled in such a short amount of time! Don't forget, the secret of a smooth trip is maintenance of that precious vehicle of yours!

The Gift

The gift I give myself,
Is the greatest I will ever know.
The gift from the heart, the gift from the soul
Is the one I will never outgrow.

This gift cannot be broken.
It cannot be bought or sold.
It is not a material token.
It is more valuable than gold.

This gift will last forever
For it is like the sea.
Strong and powerful, yet peaceful and clear,
The gift I give is "ME"!

This gift is a promise
I made long ago.
I did not know then,
How its value would grow.

It is kept far away
Where the world cannot see.
This gift it is personal,
So precious to me.

It is opened each year,
A part of my celebration.
Then re-wrapped and hidden,
Without hesitation.

My gift will be with me,
As I complete this life's journey...
The only regret I have today?
Fear delayed my gift's delivery!

Melonie Heaton

Part Three

Master Mechanic's
Tool Kit

Substitute Healthier Foods

Item	Substitute
butter/margarine	fat-free butter
Half & Half /creamer	nonfat varieties or canned evaporated skim milk
cheese	nonfat or low-fat. Soy cheese is best!
peanut butter	reduced-fat or soy
cream cheese	nonfat or low-fat varieties
sour cream	nonfat or plain nonfat yogurt
mayo	low-fat or nonfat, or nonfat ranch dressing or nonfat cream cheese or nonfat plain yogurt
cottage cheese (regular)	nonfat or low-fat varieties
whole milk	skim milk or 1% milk or canned evaporated skim milk
buttermilk	nonfat powdered buttermilk, reconstituted
regular yogurt	nonfat, artificially sweetened
ice cream	nonfat or nonfat, no-sugar-added or nonfat frozen yogurt
pudding	nonfat, artificially sweetened, made with skim milk
regular pasta (white flour)	spelt grain or whole wheat or corn or quinoa
white rice	short- or long-grain brown rice, wild rice or brown basmati rice
canned soups	choose low-fat varieties
ham	turkey ham, low-fat
bacon/sausage	turkey bacon/sausage or try vegetable or soy-based products
sugar	Barley Malt, fruit sweet, brown rice syrup or aspartame
flavored instant hot cereal	quick cooking plain, and flavor your own with fruit and/or cinnamon

salad dressings	nonfat or make your own
ground beef	extra lean, or substitute extra lean ground turkey or frozen vegetarian burger crumbles
baking chocolate squares	3 Tbsp. cocoa dissolved in a bit of water or skim milk, per square
eggs	egg whites or fat-free egg substitute
pie crust	egg roll or won ton wrappers, or phyllo dough
long-cook hot cereal	leftover short-grain brown rice with sweetener, cinnamon, applesauce or fruit
chili canned	choose low-fat or vegetarian fat-free or low-fat or turkey chili—not chicken!
canned beans (e.g., baked)	choose low-fat or fat-free
chocolate chips	carob chips
granola bars/toaster pastries	fat-free, fruit sweetened from the health food store or natural foods section of your store
whipped cream/topping	choose fat-free
jams and jellies	choose fruit spread or puréed fruit or applesauce or nonfat fruit flavored cream cheese
pizza crust	make your own nonfat or use whole wheat pitas or extra large low-fat or nonfat tortillas
regular tortillas	choose nonfat or reduced-fat
lunch meats	choose very low-fat or nonfat
regular refried beans	choose fat-free, vegetarian
cream sauces	use canned evaporated skim milk thickened with a solution of corn starch and water.
fats in baked goods	substitute instant pudding mix (nonfat) egg substitute, puréed low-fat cottage cheese or fruit-based fat substitute
tortilla chips	choose baked varieties
canned tuna in oil	choose water-pack tuna
potato chips	some baked varieties are excellent
granola	choose low-fat or nonfat, or make your own!

raisin bran	purchase sugar-free bran flakes and toss a few raisins on top to reduce sugar content!
meat or vegetable broth	choose fat-free or very low-fat
gravies	make your own with evaporated skim milk and broth, thickened with cornstarch and water!
sundried tomatoes	purchase dry and reconstitute in hot water
oils for cookware	spray oil or fat-free broth

Reading Your Fuel Gauge

Caloric Need Calculations

These calculations are provided to give you a ballpark caloric need for your age, based on your height, weight, age and activity level (A.L.). To be sure your fuel gauge is set correctly, please refer back to the chapter entitled "Fuel-Style Overhaul Time" to learn how to calculate your own caloric need.

Weight	A. L. 1	A. L. 2	A. L. 3	A. L. 4
140	1500	1700	2000	2400
150	1630	1830	2130	2530
170	1890	2090	2390	2790
185	2085	2285	2585	2985
200	2280	2480	2780	3180
220	2540	2740	3040	3440
240	2800	3000	3300	3700
260	3060	3260	3560	3960
280	3320	3520	3820	4220
300	3580	3780	4080	4480
320	3840	4040	4340	4740
340	4100	4300	4600	5000
360	4360	4560	4860	5260
380	4620	4820	5120	5520
400	4880	5080	5380	5780
420	5140	5340	5640	6040
450	5530	5730	6030	6430
475	5855	6055	6355	6755
500	6180	6380	6680	7080

There is extra space on the next page for calculating your fuel needs as explained in the chapter titled, "Fuel-Style Overhaul Time!"

Calculate your fuel needs.

Base = <u>1500</u>

For each 10 lb. increase in weight over 140 lbs., add 130 calories:

+_____

(Your body weight minus 140 lbs. divided by 10 x 130)

Add the factor for your activity level: (0, 200, 500 or 900)

+_____

Your fuel need is 200 less to 200 calories more

than this number: =_____

Base = <u>1500</u>

For each 10 lb. increase in weight over 140 lbs., add 130 calories:

+_____

(Your body weight minus 140 lbs. divided by 10 x 130)

Add the factor for your activity level: (0, 200, 500 or 900)

+_____

Your fuel need is 200 less to 200 calories more

than this number: =_____

Base = <u>1500</u>

For each 10 lb. increase in weight over 140 lbs., add 130 calories:

+_____

(Your body weight minus 140 lbs. divided by 10 x 130)

Add the factor for your activity level: (0, 200, 500 or 900)

+_____

Your fuel need is 200 less to 200 calories more

than this number: =_____

Calculating the miles per gallon

What is a serving?

We have provided you serving sizes for many foods that do not typically have labels.

Remember, for our purposes, one serving of protein = 12–16 grams (about 70–100 calories). One serving of carbohydrate also = 12–16 grams (about 100 calories). When reading labels, especially of mixed/convenience foods, look at the total protein and carbohydrate counts to determine the number of servings of each. Limit fats to no more than 30 percent of your total daily calories, preferably less but never below 10 percent. Limit sweets and simple carbohydrates. Try to consume about two servings of carbohydrate for every one serving of protein. Select foods from all of the food groups, making sure you get at least two servings of nonfat or low-fat dairy, two to three servings of fruit and three to five servings of vegetables at a minimum each day. Balance. Balance. Balance! Adjust carbohydrates upwards if you are lacking energy or are hungry more often than every two to three hours.

Protein: 70–100 calories per serving!

Very lean meats, poultry, fish and eggs

1 serving:
¼ chicken breast, boneless, skinless (1½ ounces). ½ breast = 2 protein servings
1 chicken thigh, no skin
2 chicken wings, no skin
1½ oz. turkey, roasted, light or dark meat, skin not eaten
2 eggs (Fat Alert!)
4–5 egg whites
1½ oz. lean roast beef
2 oz. lean beef steak or stew meat
2 oz. extra-lean ground beef
2 oz. lean pork roast or chops
2½ oz. cured or smoked ham (Fat Alert!)

5 slices of bacon, cooked (Fat Alert!)
2 oz. lamb chop (about ½ chop), lean (Fat Alert!)
1½ oz. lean veal
3 strips of venison jerky (about 4 inch-long pieces)
3 oz. of liver (Fat Alert!)
2½–3 frankfurters, traditional type (Major Fat Alert!)
2 turkey frankfurters
3 oz. of most white fish (flounder, sole, halibut)
2½ oz. of trout, salmon, swordfish or tuna steak
2 oz. canned, water-pack tuna
3 oz. clams, shrimp, crab, lobster or scallops
4 oz. of mussels
5 oz. of cooked oysters
8 oz. of raw oysters
1½ oz. of cooked snails

Carbohydrates: About 100 calories per serving

Breads

1 medium bagel = 2 servings
1 large bagel (like from the chain stores) = 4 servings
1 medium biscuit
1 slice of French bread (less than 1 oz. per slice)
½–1½ slices multi-grain bread (Read the labels! Some have lots of fat and calories!)
1 medium pita bread = 2 servings
1 slice of white bread
1½ oz. of cornbread
1 medium crumpet
½ English muffin, plain
½ sourdough roll
½ hamburger or hot dog bun
½ soft white dinner roll
2 taco shells (Fat Alert!)
2 tortillas (not fried)

Fruits

1 small apple
½ cup unsweetened applesauce
3 raw apricots

1 medium peach
½ medium banana
1–1½ cup raw berries
1 cup cantaloupe or other melon
¾ cup raw cherries
¾ cup raw grapefruit or orange sections
½ cup grapes
½ mango
1 nectarine
1 cup papaya
½ medium pear
¾ cup raw pineapple
2 plums
⅓ cup raisins or most any dried fruit
½ cup unsweetened fruit juice
⅓ cup sorbet

Vegetables
1 small artichoke
2 cups cooked asparagus
½ cup cooked lima beans
1½ cups cooked green beans
1 cup cooked beets
1½ cup cooked broccoli
1 cup cooked brussels sprouts
4 cups raw cabbage
2 cups cooked cabbage
2 medium carrots, raw
1 cup cooked carrots
2 cups cooked cauliflower
3 cups raw cauliflower
12–15 medium stalks of raw celery
3 cups cooked greens
½ large or 1 small ear of corn, cooked
⅓ cup cooked corn
3 cups raw cucumber, sliced
2 cups cooked eggplant
1 head of lettuce
2 cups cooked mushrooms

4 cups raw mushroom slices
1 cup cooked okra
1 cup cooked onions
1 large raw onion
½ cup green peas, cooked or raw
2 whole sweet green peppers, raw
2 cups chopped green pepper, raw
2½ cups cooked green pepper
1 cups cooked pumpkin or other yellow squash
3 cups radishes, raw, sliced
1½ cups snow peas, cooked or raw
3 cups cooked summer squash
3 medium tomatoes, raw
1½ cups cooked tomatoes
⅓ cup cooked yams or sweet potatoes
4 cups zucchini
½ medium white potato, baked
½ cup mashed potatoes

Afterthoughts: Some Answers to Questions You May Have

1. *Do I need a vitamin supplement?*

There are as many opinions out there as there are vitamin and nutritional product manufacturers. In our opinion, if you are eating high-quality fuel, and balancing your fuel by consuming the minimum number of servings from each food group, you may not need a supplement. This is really yet another of your choices. It is our belief that years of abusing the body through poor nutrition and lack of exercise robs the body of the nutrients it is able to store. We do take vitamin supplements just to make sure that we are getting all of our needs met, that we are replacing those stores, and that we are giving our bodies everything possible to get healthy. If in doubt, discuss this issue with your doctor.

2. *What about all of those herbal supplements, fat burners and muscle builders out there. Do they really work?*

Keep in mind that every body is different, and what is of benefit for one person may not be of benefit to another. It is important to note that the quality of supplements varies from manufacturer to manufacturer, and you may notice a different response if you change brands. If you do stumble upon a product that appears to give you some benefit, stick with the same brand and take it consistently, according to the label directions. Again, talk this over with your health-care provider before taking any new supplement, herb or medication.

The nutritional supplement industry is booming. It is full of products that most people either don't need or don't understand. Some herbal products in particular will react in a way similar to prescription medications. These products are not regulated for the most part. We have tried to teach you that anything you put into your body should not be taken lightly. Nutritional supplements are no exception. Do your research. Understand how each is used, and make educated decisions about what you will put into your body!

3. *I am eating right, moving my body and I think I'm giving my body what it needs, when it needs it. I keep adjusting my fuel intake but I am hungry all the time, really hungry, and usually within an hour or two after I eat. What am I doing wrong?*

Depending on how long you have been using BodyLogic, and how long you have been abusing your body through years of starvation and inactivity, your hunger may be just your body's response to leaving starvation mode. Your increased hunger will not last for long. Eat only when hungry. If you are balancing your meals, and if you are eating more complex carbohydrates than simple carbohydrates, then you may have a medical problem. And you should check with your doctor.

4. *I have been using BodyLogic for over two months and so far I don't see any real changes. I have not lost weight or inches, and my activity program is not getting any easier. Does this mean that BodyLogic won't work for me?*

Again, much depends upon how long you have been overfat and inactive. It can take several months for your body to reverse the trend of starvation. First of all, you should not still be using your scale! Second, evaluate how often you are doing your activity sessions. If these sessions occur more than once a day, or if you are doing them daily and you are over age thirty-five, you may be overdoing it. Listen to your body. Does it hurt anywhere? If so, that is a strong indication that you are overdoing things. Third, revaluate your caloric need. Refer back to some of the food chapters. Adjust your caloric intake up or down 100 or 200 calories then sit tight for another four to six weeks. Then revaluate things again. The hardest part to achieving a successful lifestyle change is to learn how to listen to your body, and to interpret the messages it is giving you. Lots of trial and error now will help you to become successful later. Time is on your side. You are not in a race. Your goal should be health, not losing a certain number of pounds or inches. Just eat right, move your body, and listen to your body. It will take care of the rest as nature intended.

5. *All of the food calculations, menu planning and decisions to be made at the grocery store seem really overwhelming. Isn't there an easier way?*

Our question for you is this. Are you trying to make too many changes all at once? Focus on one thing at a time. Start with trying to keep your total caloric intake at 30 percent fat or less. We have given you simple tools to evaluate your progress with this. Once you have achieved this goal, you can either reduce that fat content down, or start focusing on something else, like making sure you are getting enough protein or are limiting your intake of refined sugar. One small step at a time, many small steps over a long period of time, will make the transition into your new lifestyle much easier!

My Progress Chart for the year _____

	Jan.	Feb.	Mar.	Apr.	May
Chest					
Bust					
Below bust					
Waist					
7" below waist					
Hip					
Right thigh					
Left thigh					
Right calf					
Left calf					
Right upper arm					
Left upper arm					
Other					
Dress size					
Weight					
Totals:					
Inches lost					
Pounds lost					

My Progress Chart for the year _____

Jun.	Jul.	Aug.	Sept.	Oct.	Nov.	Dec.

My Activity Record

	Week 1	Week 2	Week 3	Week 4	Week 5	Week 6
Activity 1						
Time						
Distance						
Activity 2						
Time						
Distance						
Activity 3						
Time						
Distance						
Activity 4						
Time						
Distance						
Resting pulse						
Blood pressure						

My Activity Record

Week 6	Week 7	Week 8	Week 9	Week 10	Week 11	Week 12

Here's how to contact us!

BodyLogic LLC

Phone: 1-800-831-8835   Fax: 503-661-7501
Snail Mail: 15 N.E. 181st. Ave., Portland, OR 97230-6659
E-mail: BodyLo1997@aol.com
Visit Our Web Site: http://www.BodyLogic-Is-For-Me.com

You may order additional books with credit card by calling: 1-(800) 356-9315

Snail mail/fax merchandise order form:

Qty.	Item	Price Each	Total
_____	**Extra-length (120-inch) tape measure**	$3.50	_____
_____	**BodyLogic bumper sticker**	$3.50	
	"BURNING FAT, FEELING WOW! BODYLOGIC TAUGHT ME HOW!"		_____
_____	**BodyLogic Newsletter,** issued quarterly.		
	One-year subscription	$12.95	_____
_____	**BodyLogic Club Membership**	$40.00	_____
	Membership includes the newsletter and a 10% discount on all merchandise, seminars and workshops. New members will receive a bumper sticker and a tape measure.		

Total order _____

Fax/electronic orders payable by credit card only.
Send order to: (please print)

Ms/Mrs/Mr _____
          First   Middle initial   Last name

Address: _____,_____
        Street   City   State   Zip

Payment method: check/charge

(MC or Visa) card #: _____Exp. date:_____

Name as printed on credit card: _____

Signature (required) _____

Phone number: (   )_____